FOOT FUNCTION
a programmed text

FOOT FUNCTION
a programmed text

Michael O. Seibel, D.O., D.P.M.

Diplomate, American Board of Podiatric Orthopedics

Associate Clinical Professor of Podiatric Medicine
University of Osteopathic Medicine and Health Sciences
College of Podiatric Medicine and Surgery
Des Moines, Iowa

Formerly
Assistant Professor of Biomechanics
California College of Podiatric Medicine
San Francisco, California

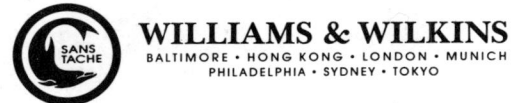

WILLIAMS & WILKINS
BALTIMORE · HONG KONG · LONDON · MUNICH
PHILADELPHIA · SYDNEY · TOKYO

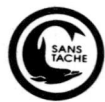

Editor: Jonathan W. Pine, Jr.
Associate Editor: Linda Napora
Copy Editor: Janis Oppelt
Design: JoAnne Janowiak
Illustration Planning: Lorraine Wrzosek
Production: Raymond E. Reter
Cover Design: Michael O. Seibel

Copyright © 1988
Williams & Wilkins
428 East Preston Street
Baltimore, MD 21202, USA

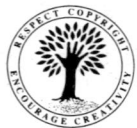

All rights reserved. This book is protected by copyright. No part of this book may be reproduced in any form or by any means, including photocopying, or utilized by any information storage and retrieval system without written permission from the copyright owner.

Printed in the United States of America

Library of Congress Cataloging-in-Publication Data

Seibel, Michael O.
  Foot function.

  Includes index.
  1. Foot—Programmed instruction. 2. Foot—Diseases—Programmed instruction. 3. Human mechanics—Programmed instruction. I. Title. [DNLM: 1. Foot—physiology—programmed instruction. WE 18 S457f]
  RD563.S39 1988   612'.98   87-23125
  ISBN 0-683-07651-5

This book is dedicated to my family: to Kerry for her unfaltering faith, support, encouragement, and vision; to Jacob, for putting things in perspective; to Barry, for his lucid inspiration; to Joe, for standing with us; and to Carol and Dr. Aron Seibel for their guidance and support.

Foreword

Podiatric biomechanics is a simultaneously frustrating and rewarding area of clinical medicine. Understanding opens new and exciting avenues of approach in the treatment of a host of lower extremity pathological conditions. With greater knowledge comes enhanced ability to initiate increasingly efficient treatment regimens that alter foot and leg mechanics.

Until now, a void has existed between the theoretical knowledge of normal and abnormal foot and leg mechanics and their clinical recognition, evaluation, and treatment. Fortunately, however, the longstanding need for a text to bridge the gap between mechanical theory and observable and reproducible clinical experiences has finally been met in *Foot Function: A Programmed Text*. Dr. Seibel has clearly established the parameters for becoming comfortable with the classic functioning of lower extremity biomechanics and effectively applying these guidelines to common clinical situations.

Foot Function, by virtue of its own inherent mechanics of presenting a programmed concept of understanding, further allows the student to think in mechanical terms and begin to evaluate problems in a precise and ordered fashion. This book will enable those with only a basic and rudimentary knowledge of biomechanics to reach a level of clear understanding and to apply the principles to the common day-to-day pathologies we all treat.

This book immediately establishes itself as a classic work in our overall education in the principles and techniques necessary for proper evaluation of musculoskeletal pathologies. All students—past, present and future—will benefit from reading and rereading this well-thought-out and clinically significant work.

Ronald L. Valmassy, D.P.M.
Professor and Former Chairman
Department of Biomechanics
California College of Podiatric Medicine
San Francisco, California

Preface

This text is designed to introduce functional biomechanics of the foot in an enhanced retention format. Hopefully, this type of learning experience will be a useful adjunct in the didactic presentation of foot biomechanics. Additionally, it should be serviceable as a tool for the practitioner to help expand or reinforce previously existing knowledge in this specialty area.

The goal of this book is to provide the reader with an understanding of foot function in the normal and common pathologic states. To this end, the reader is exposed to the fundamental considerations of foot function as well as clinical considerations such as the biomechanical examination.

In the format employed in this book, the answer to the question or blank is in the left margin next to the frame immediately following. Thus, by simply covering the entire portion of the page below the statement being assessed, the eye of the reader should not experience any temptation to roam to the answer prematurely. After arriving at a response, the reader should move the cover sheet down (just past the next frame) to see if the answer is correct, and, if so, continue with the next frame (beside the correct response to the previous one). If an incorrect response has been given, the reader should go back to the frame(s) explaining the subject under consideration and proceed forward from that point.

In this manner, the reader should develop a sound and rational command of the material being presented. It is suggested that one and only one chapter should be completed at a sitting. By completing more material, long-term retention may be diminished. By completing less than one chapter, the logical train of thought is broken, again potentially sacrificing retention.

Foot function is conceptually complex. It is the intent of this book to present this subject in a manner that is educationally valid and intellectually comfortable.

Enjoy your learning experience!

Acknowledgments

I would like to express my very special appreciation to Ronald Valmassy, D.P.M., who gave me the initial encouragement and support to embark upon this project.

Additionally, thanks are due to J. Leonard Azneer, Ph.D., and Leonard A. Levy, D.P.M., M.P.H., for their encouragement of this undertaking.

Also, I would like to thank my editor, Jonathan W. Pine, Jr., and my associate editor, Linda Napora, for their help and support throughout this book's conception and publication.

Contents

Foreword by Ronald L. Valmassy, D.P.M. vii
Preface ix
Acknowledgments x

Chapter 1	Introductory Nomenclature	1
Chapter 2	Joint Axes and Motions	15
Chapter 3	Joint Axes and Motions—Foot	21
Chapter 4	Overview of the Gait Cycle	41
Chapter 5	Subtalar Joint Function in Open and Closed Kinetic Chain	51
Chapter 6	Normal Subtalar Joint Function in the Gait Cycle	59
Chapter 7	Subtalar Joint—Open Kinetic Chain Measurement and Neutral Position Calculation	69
Chapter 8	Factors Affecting Rearfoot Position	81
Chapter 9	Rearfoot and Subtalar Joint: Closed Kinetic Chain Measurement and Evaluation	97
Chapter 10	Mini-Workbook: Subtalar Joint Case Histories (Calculations and Interpretations)	109
Chapter 11	Effects of Rearfoot Pathology on the Gait Cycle	123
Chapter 12	Normal Midtarsal Joint Function and Measurement	135
Chapter 13	Normal Midtarsal Joint Function in the Gait Cycle	149

Chapter 14	Midtarsal Joint Deformity and Its Effects on the Gait Cycle	165
Chapter 15	Function of the First and Fifth Rays and the Metatarsaphalangeal Joints	187
Chapter 16	First Ray Pathology and Its Effects on the Gait Cycle	201
Chapter 17	Biomechanical Examination—Non-Weight bearing Assessment	213
Chapter 18	Biomechanical Examination—Weight bearing Assessment	237
Appendix I	Signs and Symptoms Associated with Biomechanical Pathology in the Foot	253
Appendix II	Criteria for Normalcy in the Lower Extremity	255
Appendix III	Effects in the Foot Secondary to Abnormal Propulsive STJ Pronation	256
	Glossary	257
	Index	263

CHAPTER
1

Introductory Nomenclature

- body planes
- single plane motions of the foot
- single plane positions of the foot
- triplane motions of the foot
- triplane positions of the foot
- fixed structural positions of the foot

1-1
In order to define body motion and position, the three body planes are used for points of reference. These body planes are the *sagittal, frontal,* and *transverse* planes (Fig. 1.1).

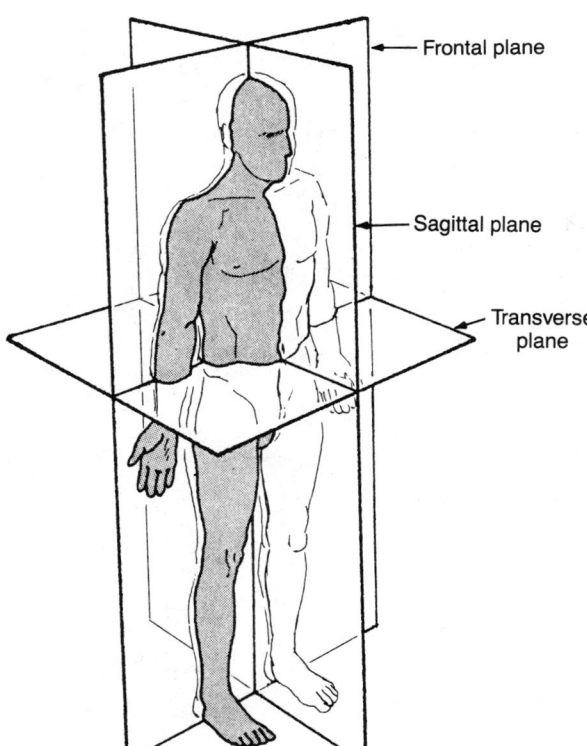

Figure 1.1.
The three body planes. From Inman VT, Ralston HJ, Todd, F: *Human Walking.* Baltimore, Williams & Wilkins, 1981, p 34.

1-2
The three body planes—sagittal, frontal, and transverse—are used as points of _____ in defining body motion and position.

reference

1-3
The *sagittal* plane is one of the _____ body planes and divides the body into right and left portions.

three

1-4
The *frontal* plane is perpendicular to the sagittal plane. The frontal plane divides the body into a front portion and a back portion, whereas the *sagittal* plane divides the body into _____ and _____ portions.

right, left

1-5
The plane which separates the body into front and back portions is the _____ plane.

frontal

1-6
The last of the three body planes is the *transverse* plane. It is perpendicular to the other two planes (i.e., the _____ and _____ planes) and separates the body into upper and lower portions.

sagittal, frontal

1-7
The three body planes are the _____, _____, and _____.

sagittal, frontal, transverse

1-8
The plane which separates the body into front and back portions is a _____ plane.

The plane which separates the body into right and left portions is a _____ plane.

The plane which separates the body into top and bottom portions is a _____ plane.

frontal, sagittal, transverse

1-9
If a motion occurs parallel to (or within) a particular body plane, for example a sagittal plane, it would be called a sagittal plane motion (Fig. 1.2).

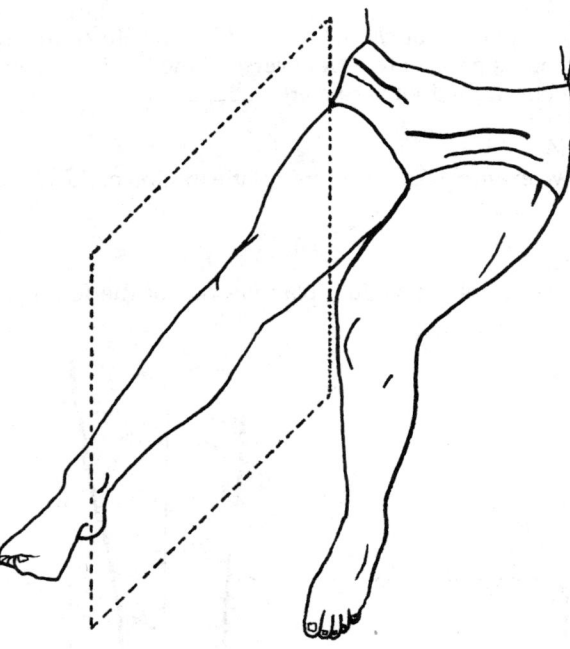

Figure 1.2.
Knee flexion occurs parallel to a sagittal plane and is therefore a sagittal plane motion.

1-10
If a motion occurs parallel to a *transverse* plane, it would be called a ____Trans____ plane motion.

transverse

1-11
Knee flexion occurs parallel to a sagittal plane and is therefore classified as a _____ plane motion.

sagittal

1-12
An example of transverse plane *motion* is abduc*tion* in which the foot (or part of the foot) is rotated externally while remaining parallel to a _____ plane (Fig. 1.3).

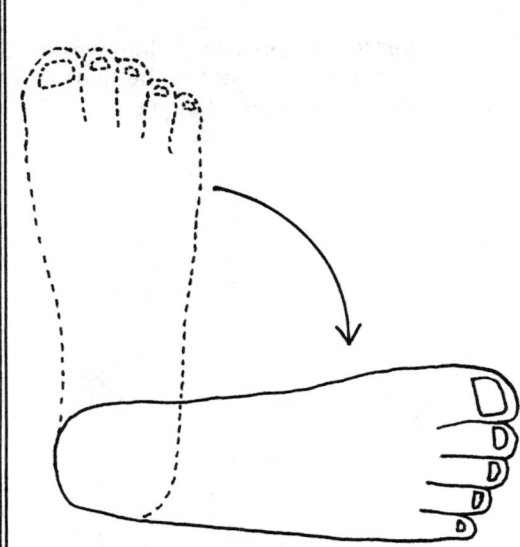

Figure 1.3.
Foot abduction.

transverse

1-13
The opposite of *ab*duction is *ad*duction. In *ad*duction, the foot also remains parallel to a transverse plane but is rotated *internally*. In *ab*duction, the foot is rotated _____.

externally

1-14
Two examples of transverse plane motion of the foot are _____ and _____.

abduction, adduction

1-15
An example of sagittal plane *motion* of the foot is dorsiflex*ion* (Fig. 1.4).

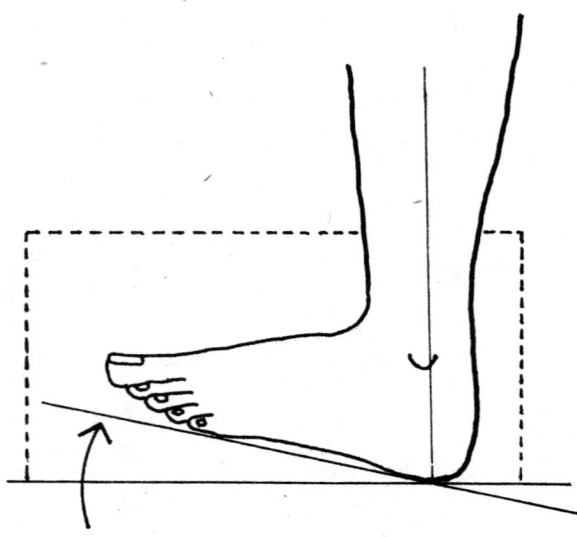

Figure 1.4.
Dorsiflexion occurs parallel to a sagittal plane.

1-16
In *dorsiflexion*, the distal part of the foot (or part of the foot) moves parallel to a _____ plane, toward the tibia.

sagittal

1-17
Plantarflexion is the opposite of dorsiflexion. In plantarflexion, the distal part of the foot (or part of the foot) moves (*away from/toward*) the tibia, parallel to a sagittal plane.

1: INTRODUCTORY NOMENCLATURE

away from

1-18
In the normal foot, the reference point for a dorsiflex*ed* or plantarflex*ed position* is a transverse plane which runs through the heel. If the foot is positioned below this transverse plane, it is said to be plantarflexed; above this transverse plane, it is said to be _____ (Fig. 1.5).

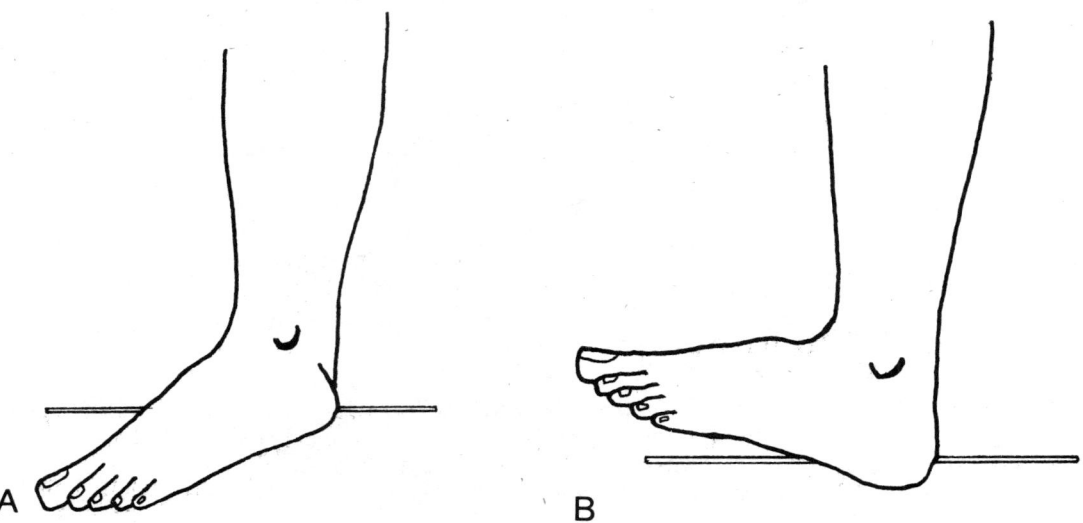

Figure 1.5.
A, A plantarflexed position. B, This foot is positioned *above* the transverse plane.

dorsiflexed

1-19
Dorsiflex*ed* refers to *position*. Dorsiflex*ion* refers to _____.

motion

1-20
The reference point in a normal foot for judging a position to be dorsiflexed or plantarflexed is a _____ plane which runs through the heel.

transverse

1-21
If a foot is in a 10° dorsiflexed attitude (i.e., angulated 10° above the transverse plane) and moves to a 15° plantarflexed attitude (i.e., angulated 15° below the tranverse plane), the *motion* that it has gone through would be classified as _____.

plantarflexion

1-22
If a foot is in a 15° plantarflexed attitude and moves to a 10° dorsiflexed attitude, the motion would be classified as _____.

dorsiflexion

1-23
If a foot is in a 15° plantarflexed attitude and moves to a 10° plantarflexed attitude (Fig. 1.6), the motion it has gone through would be classified as ___DF___.

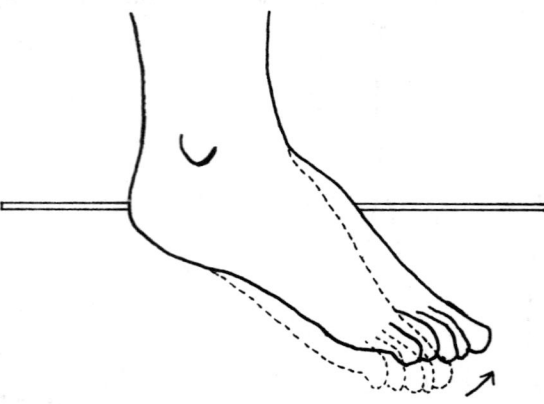

Figure 1.6.

dorsiflexion

1-24
The reason that the answer to frame 1-23 is dorsiflexion is that, even though the foot ends up in a plantarflexed position (judged relative to a transverse plane running through the heel), it is *moving (away from/toward)* the tibia.

toward

1-25
So then, a foot in a 15° dorsiflexed attitude moving to a 10° dorsiflexed attitude exhibits the *motion* of _____.

plantarflexion

1-26
Two sagittal plane motions of the foot are _____ and _____. The foot's distal aspect or part moves *away from* the tibia in the motion of _____.

dorsiflexion, plantarflexion, plantarflexion

1-27
Two transverse plane motions of the foot are ___ab___ and _____.

abduction, adduction

1-28
In abduction, the foot or part of the foot is rotated _____, thus moving the distal aspect of the foot or part *(away from/toward)* the midline of the body.

externally, away from

1-29
The two frontal plane motions of the foot are inversion and eversion. By definition, these motions occur ___parallel___ to a frontal plane.

parallel

1-30
With inversion, the foot or part of the foot moves parallel to a _____ plane so as to tilt the foot or part more toward the midline of the body.

frontal

1-31
As you might guess, with eversion, the foot or part of the foot moves parallel to a frontal plane so as to tilt the foot or part further (*away from/toward*) the midline of the body.

away from

1-32
The two frontal plane *motions* of the foot are _____ and _____.
The two *positions* of the foot relative to the frontal plane are called *inverted* and *everted*.

inversion, eversion

1-33
A foot or part of a foot is said to be *inverted* when it is tilted parallel to a ___frontal___ plane so that the plantar surface of the foot or part faces *toward the midline of the body* and *away from a transverse body plane* (or away from some other specified reference point).

frontal

1-34
A foot or part of the foot is said to be everted when it is tilted parallel to a frontal plane so that the plantar surface faces away from the midline of the body and away from a transverse body plane (Fig. 1.7).

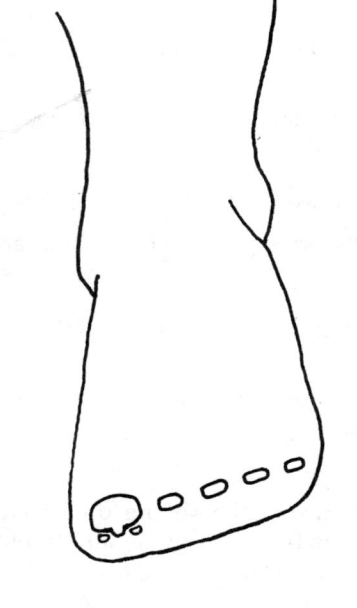

Figure 1.7.
An everted position.

1-35
Given that both an inverted foot and an everted foot must face away from a transverse body plane, the difference between the two is in their orientation to the _____ of the body.

midline

1-36
The everted foot faces (*away from/toward*) the midline of the body and away from a transverse body plane.

away from	**1-37** An inverted foot faces (*away from/toward*) the midline of the body and away from a transverse body plane.
toward	**1-38** Both inverted and everted feet refer to positions which are parallel to a _____ plane.
frontal	**1-39** If a foot goes from a 4° everted position to a 2° inverted position, the *motion* that has occurred is classified as _____.
inversion	**1-40** If a foot goes from a 5° inverted position to a 3° everted position, the *motion* that has occurred is classified as _____.
eversion	**1-41** If a foot goes from a 5° inverted position to a 2° inverted position, the motion that has occurred is classified as _____. (HINT: Remember the difference between position and motion.)
eversion	**1-42** To review, the two frontal plane *motions* of the foot are _____ and _____. The two frontal plane *positions* of the foot are _____ and _____.
inversion, eversion, inverted, everted	**1-43** The foot's two sagittal plane *motions* are _____ and _____. The foot's two sagittal plane *positions* are _____ and _____.
dorsiflexion, plantar- flexion, dorsiflexed, plantarflexed	**1-44** The two transverse plane *motions* of the foot are _____ and _____. The two transverse plane *positions* of the foot are _____ and _____.
abduction, adduction, abducted, adducted	**1-45** There are two motions of the foot which include simultaneous movement in the frontal, sagittal, and transverse planes. These motions are called *pronation* and *supination*. By definition, they are *triplane motions*.
	1-46 Pronation is a _____ motion composed of abduction, dorsiflexion, and eversion.

1: INTRODUCTORY NOMENCLATURE

triplane

1-47
From that, you may extrapolate that a pronated position is one in which the foot is abducted, dorsiflexed, and _____ (Fig. 1.8).

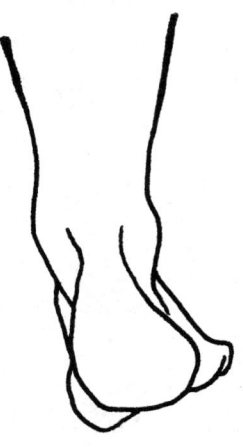

Figure 1.8.
A pronated position.

1-48
In supination, the foot undergoes motion composed of adduction, plantarflexion, and inversion. Hence, supination is the opposite of _____.

everted

pronation

1-49
It follows, from the definition of supination, that a supinated position is one in which the foot is _____, _____, and inverted (Fig. 1.9).

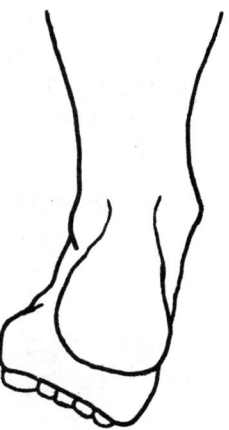

Figure 1.9.
A supinated position.

adducted, plantar-flexed

1-50
Since it is difficult to clinically measure a triplane motion (specifically at the subtalar joint), frontal plane motion is used as an *index* to measure triplane motion (specifically at the _____ joint).

subtalar	**1-51** The positions of the foot studied thus far are just that—positions. In the case of a *fixed structural position*, words are used which denote just that—a fixed _____ position.
structural	**1-52** *Adductus* denotes a fixed structural position in which the foot is held _____.
adducted	**1-53** *Ab*ductus denotes a _____ _____ _____ in which the foot is held abducted.
fixed structural position	**1-54** Apparently, the suffix "*us*" is associated with positions which are _____ _____ positions.
fixed structural	**1-55** If the foot or part of the foot is *rotated externally* (parallel to a transverse plane) with its distal aspect facing *away from the midline* and the position is a *fixed structural* one, the foot or part of the foot is said to be in an *abductus* position.
abductus	**1-56** If one observes the foot or its part to be in a *fixed structural position* in which it is *rotated internally* (parallel with a transverse plane) with its distal aspect facing *toward the midline*, the foot or part is said to be in an *adductus* position.
adductus	**1-57** The *motion* in which the foot or part is rotated externally, with its distal aspect facing away from the midline, and in which the foot or part remains parallel with a transverse plane is called _____.
abduction	**1-58** The *position* that the foot is in when it is rotated internally (parallel with a transverse plane) and in which the distal aspect of the foot or part faces toward the midline is called _____.
adducted	**1-59** Two triplane motions of the foot are _____ and _____. The corresponding positions would then be _____ and _____.
pronation, supination, pronated, supinated	**1-60** If a foot is in *adductus*, it is in a _____ structural position where it is _____. If a foot or part of a foot was adducted by active muscle contraction, the *motion* that it would go through would be classified as _____.
fixed, adducted, adduction	**1-61** In *ab*ductus, the foot is in a fixed structural position where it is _____. In other words, the foot or its part is in a fixed structural position in which it is rotated _____, parallel to a *Tv* plane, and in which the distal aspect faces (*away from*/*toward*) the midline.

1: INTRODUCTORY NOMENCLATURE

1-62
There are two frontal plane fixed positions which the foot may assume relative to the inverted and everted positions. Respectively, they are *varus* and *valgus*.

abducted, externally, transverse, away from

1-63
The fixed structural position that the foot or its part assumes if it is in an inverted position is classified as _____.

varus

1-64
A fixed structural position in which the foot or part of the foot appears *everted* is classified as _____.

valgus

1-65
There are two fixed structural positions of the foot which are relative to the sagittal plane position. The two sagittal plane *positions* are _____ and _____.

dorsiflexed, plantarflexed

1-66
If a foot is in a fixed structural position in which it appears dorsiflexed, it is classified as a *talipes calcaneus* type foot (only the calcaneus contacts the ground). *Talipes* refers to any deformity of the foot which involves the talus (Fig. 1.10).

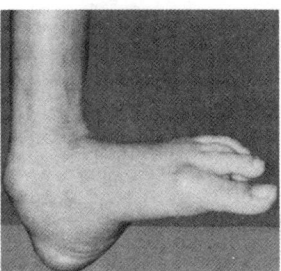

Figure 1.10. Talipes calcaneus. From Salter RB: *Textbook of Disorders and Injuries of the Musculoskeletal System.* ed 2. Baltimore, Williams & Wilkins, 1983, p 47.

1-67
Talipes calcaneus refers to a _____ _____ position in which the foot is positioned (*above/below*) a transverse plane which runs through the heel.

FOOT FUNCTION: A PROGRAMMED TEXT

fixed structural, above

1-68
If the foot is positioned below a transverse plane which runs through the heel in an exclusively sagittal plane deviation (i.e., *dorsiflexed/plantarflexed*), it is known as a *talipes equinus* foot type. Equinus comes from the Latin word meaning horselike. In this context, it refers to the hooflike appearance of the foot (Fig. 1.11).

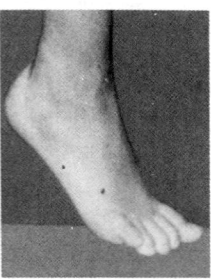

Figure 1.11. Talipes equinus. From Salter RB: *Textbook of Disorders and Injuries of the Musculoskeletal System.* ed 3. Baltimore, Williams & Wilkins, 1983, p 47.

plantarflexed

1-69
So, the two fixed structural positions of the foot that are exclusive deviations in the sagittal plane are _____ _____ and _____ _____.

talipes calcaneus, talipes equinus

1-70
Talipes calcaneus refers to the the fixed structural position of the foot in which it is held _____ed.

dorsiflex(ed)

1-71
Talipes equinus refers to the _____ _____ position of the foot in which it is held _____ed.

fixed structural, plantarflex(ed)

1-72
To review, the fixed structural positions of the foot relative to the transverse plane are _____ and _____.

abductus, adductus

1-73
The two fixed structural positions of the foot that are exclusive deviations in the frontal plane are _____ and _____.

varus, valgus

1-74
The two fixed structural positions of the foot exclusively in the sagittal plane are _____ _____ and _____ _____.

talipes calcaneus, talipes equinus

1-75
The two triplane motions of the foot are _____ and supination.

pronation

1-76
Congratulations! You have successfully completed the first chapter of your programmed textbook in Foot Function!

Questions

Instructions

In each of the following questions, select the best answer after reading *all* choices. The frame(s) specified immediately following the question illustrate the concept involved either directly or by extrapolation.

1. The plane which divides the body into right and left portions is the:
   a. sagittal plane
   b. frontal plane
   c. transverse plane
   d. oblique plane
   e. tangential plane

   FRAME 1-3

2. The transverse plane is perpendicular to which of the following?
   a. sagittal plane
   b. frontal plane
   c. oblique plane
   d. a and b
   e. a, b, and c

   FRAME 1-6

3. The motion in which the foot remains parallel to the transverse plane but is rotated internally is called:
   a. inversion
   b. dorsiflexion
   c. abductus
   d. adduction
   e. eversion

   FRAME 1-13

4. In which of the following motions does the foot move parallel to the sagittal plane only?
   a. dorsiflexion
   b. plantarflexion
   c. pronation
   d. a and b
   e. a, b, and c

   FRAME 1-26, 1-45

5. The motion that occurs if a foot goes from a 7° inverted position to a 1° everted position is called:
   a. dorsiflexion
   b. plantarflexion
   c. inversion
   d. eversion
   e. abduction

   FRAME 1-40

FRAME 1-20

6. The reference point for judging a position to be dorsiflexed or plantarflexed is the sagittal plane.
   a. true
   b. false

FRAME 1-29

7. Inversion occurs:
   a. parallel to a transverse plane
   b. perpendicular to a transverse plane
   c. parallel to a sagittal plane
   d. perpendicular to a frontal plane
   e. parallel to a frontal plane

FRAME 1-33

8. When a foot is tilted parallel with a frontal plane so that the plantar surface of the foot faces *toward* the midline of the body, the foot is said to be:
   a. pronated
   b. dorsiflexed
   c. abducted
   d. inverted
   e. none of the above

FRAME 1-23

9. The motion that a foot exhibits when it goes from a 14° dorsiflexed position to an 8° dorsiflexed position is:
   a. dorsiflexion
   b. plantarflexion
   c. inversion
   d. eversion
   e. abduction

FRAME 1-65, 1-66

10. Talipes calcaneus refers to:
    a. a fixed structural position of the foot relative to the sagittal plane
    b. a deformity which involves the talus
    c. a deformity in which only the calcaneus does not touch the ground
    d. a and b
    e. a, b, and c

Answers

1. a
2. d
3. d
4. d
5. d
6. b
7. e
8. d
9. b
10. d

CHAPTER 2

Joint Axes and Motions

- motion about an axis
- rules governing motion about an axis
- one-, two-, and three-plane axes

2-1
Each of the joints of the foot possesses an *axis* around which motion occurs.

2-2
Motion in a foot joint occurs around an _____.

axis

2-3
As illustrated by a hinge, _____ occurring around an axis is *perpendicular* to that axis (Fig. 2.1).

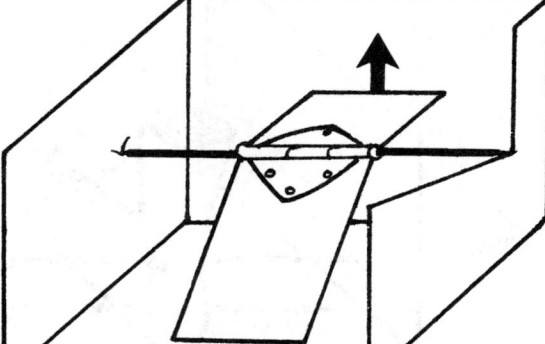

Figure 2.1.
Motion occurs perpendicular to the hinge's axis.

motion

2-4
While it is not precisely the case, let us assume for the purpose of discussion that the ankle joint's motion is pure dorsiflexion-plantarflexion (i.e., _____ plane motion), then one would correctly surmise that the joint axis is _____ to the sagittal plane (Fig. 2.2).

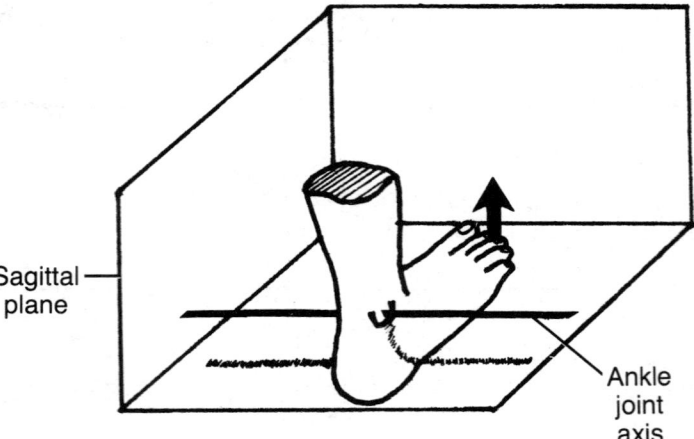

Figure 2.2.
Note that motion occurs in the sagittal plane which is perpendicular to this ankle joint axis.

sagittal, perpendicular

2-5
It is interesting to note that while the axis may be perpendicular to the sagittal plane, it can potentially be parallel to both the frontal and transverse planes (Fig. 2.3).

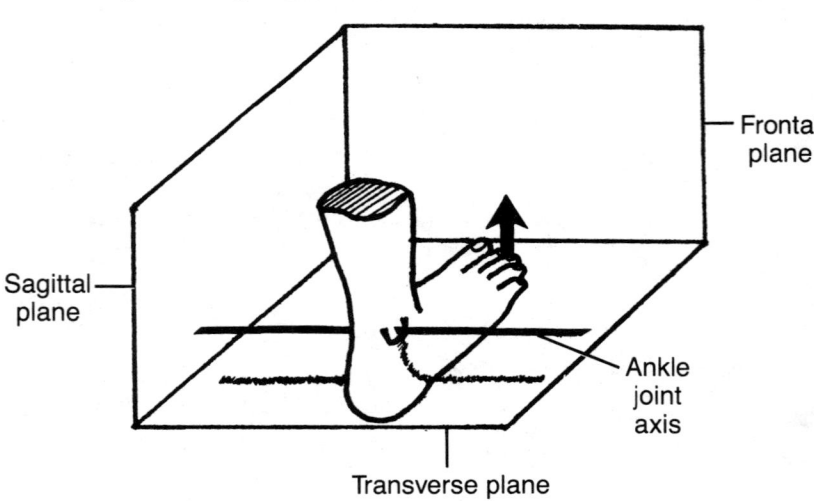

Figure 2.3.
Sagittal plane motion occurs perpendicular to the joint axis which is parallel to both the frontal and transverse planes.

2-6
If the motion occurring around a joint axis was pure inversion-eversion (i.e., frontal plane motion), one might correctly infer that the axis is potentially parallel to both the _____ and the _____ planes.

transverse, sagittal

2-7
It would seem from these mental gymnastics that a joint axis can be potentially parallel to any plane in which its motion does *not* occur.

2: JOINT AXES AND MOTIONS

2-8
If motion occurring around a joint axis was pure abduction-adduction (i.e., transverse plane motion), the axis could be parallel to both the _____ and _____ planes.

sagittal, frontal

2-9
If motion occurred around a joint axis that was both sagittal and frontal plane motion, then one might assume that the joint axis can only be parallel to one plane—the _____ plane.

transverse

2-10
Reread frame 2-9. The reason that the joint axis can only be parallel to the transverse plane is because no _____ occurred in the transverse plane.

motion

2-11
In fact, the case in frame 2-9 is pretty much the way the axis of the first ray is angulated (Fig. 2.4). Because it is practically parallel to the transverse plane, the only motion occurring is dorsiflexion-plantarflexion and _____-_____.

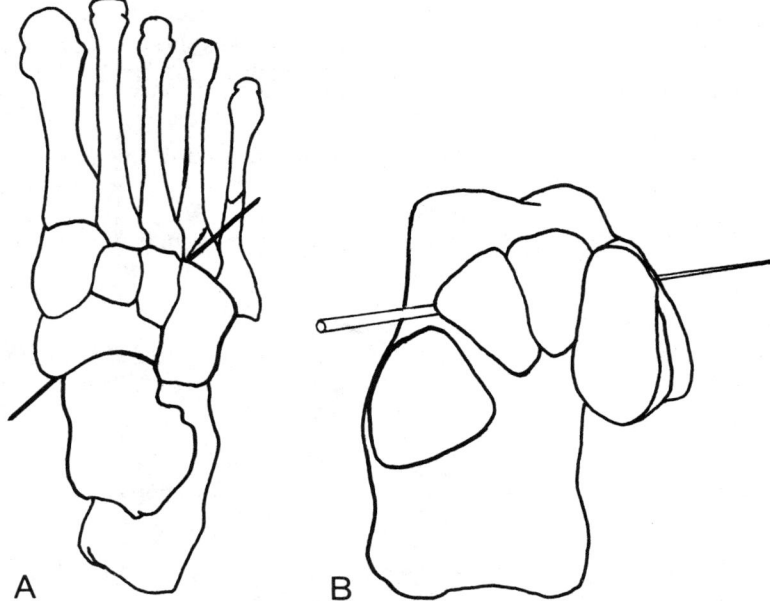

Figure 2.4. *A*, A dorsal view of the first ray's axis. *B*, A distal view (looking at the cuboid and cuneiforms) illustrating the first ray's axis.

inversion, eversion

2-12
Just to review, motion occurs _____ to the joint axis.

perpendicular

2-13
A joint axis may potentially be parallel to any plane that motion (*does/ does not*) occur in.

does not	**2-14** If motion occurs purely in only *one* plane, then the joint axis may potentially be parallel to (*one/two*) plane(s).
two	**2-15** If motion occurs purely in *two* planes, then the joint axis may potentially be parallel to (*one/two*) plane(s).
one	**2-16** It would follow that if motion occurred in all three planes, the joint axis would be parallel to (*all of them/none of them*).
none of them	**2-17** So, a motion such as pronation would indicate that the joint axis around which it occurred was an axis that was (*parallel/not parallel*) to the three body planes.
not parallel	**2-18** An axis not parallel to any of the three body planes is called a *triplane* axis because it is angulated to all three body planes.
	2-19 An axis angulated to all three body planes (i.e., not parallel with any of them) is called a _____ axis.
triplane	**2-20** Joint motion occurs around the joint's _____.
axis	**2-21** In the foot, motion occurring around the joint axis is _____ to that axis.
perpendicular	**2-22** If the motion that occurs around a joint axis is solely within (i.e., parallel to) a single plane, then the axis may be parallel to the other (*one/two*) plane(s).
two	**2-23** If motion occurs only in the transverse and sagittal planes, then the joint axis must be parallel to the _____ plane.
frontal	**2-24** On the other hand, if the joint axis is only parallel with the sagittal plane, then one would expect motion in the _____ and _____ planes.
frontal, transverse	**2-25** If supination occurred around a joint's axis, one would correctly infer that the axis was a _____ axis.
triplane	**2-26** This completes the section on joint axes and motion. Congratulations! Keep up the good work!

Questions

FRAME 2-3

1. Motion occurs _____ to a joint's axis.
   a. parallel
   b. oblique
   c. tangential
   d. perpendicular
   e. kitty-corner

FRAME 2-14

2. If a joint axis is parallel to the sagittal plane, it *cannot* be parallel to the transverse plane.
   a. always true
   b. always false
   c. only true if there is no transverse plane motion
   d. only true if there is transverse plane motion
   e. only true if there is sagittal plane motion

FRAME 2-25

3. If motion occurs *only* in the transverse and sagittal planes, that joint's axis is parallel to which of the following planes?
   a. transverse
   b. sagittal
   c. frontal
   d. a and b
   e. a, b, and c

FRAME 2-19

4. A joint axis which is a *triplane* axis is angulated to:
   a. only one body plane
   b. only two body planes
   c. all three body planes
   d. the planes with which it is parallel
   e. a and d

FRAME 2-17

5. With a triplane joint axis, motion will occur in:
   a. the sagittal plane only
   b. the transverse plane only
   c. the frontal plane only
   d. both a and b
   e. a, b, and c

6. If motion occurs in the sagittal and frontal planes around a joint axis, then that joint's axis must be parallel with the:

   a. sagittal plane
   b. frontal plane
   c. transverse plane
   d. both a and b
   e. a, b, and c

FRAME 2-11

7. If motion about a joint's axis is pure abduction-adduction, then that joint's axis *is not* parallel to the:

   a. sagittal plane
   b. frontal plane
   c. transverse plane
   d. both a and b
   e. a, b, and c

FRAME 2-4

8. A joint axis may be potentially parallel to any plane in which its motion occurs.

   a. true
   b. false

FRAME 2-7

9. The subtalar joint possesses a triplane axis. Therefore:

   a. its motion occurs in all three body planes
   b. its axis is angulated to all three body planes
   c. its axis is parallel to all three body planes
   d. a and b
   e. a and c

FRAME 2-17, 2-19

10. If a joint's axis is only parallel with the frontal plane, one would expect to see motion in the:

    a. sagittal plane only
    b. transverse plane only
    c. frontal plane only
    d. a and b
    e. a, b, and c

FRAME 2-26

Answers

1. d
2. d
3. c
4. c
5. e
6. c
7. c
8. b
9. d
10. d

CHAPTER 3

Joint Axes and Motions—Foot

- first ray axis and motion
- STJ's effect on first ray motion
- STJ's effect on distal joints
- STJ axis and motion
- fifth ray axis and motion
- central three rays axes and motions
- metatarsophalangeal joint axis and motion
- interphalangeal joint axes and motions
- midtarsal joint axes and motions

3-1
As was mentioned in Chapter 2, the first ray's axis is practically parallel only to the transverse plane (Fig. 3.1). This means that motion (*will/will not*) occur in the transverse plane.

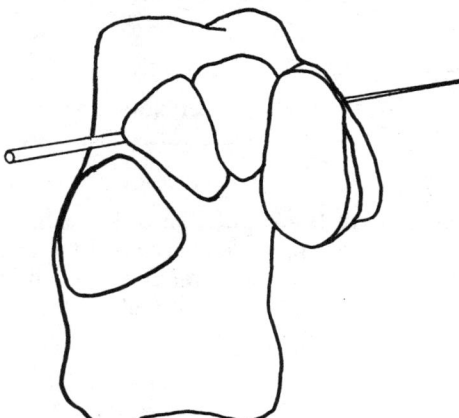

Figure 3.1.
A distal view of the first ray's axis. Note how it almost parallels the transverse plane.

will not

3-2
Since the transverse plane is the only plane that the axis parallels (for all practical purposes), one may assume that while no motion occurs in the transverse plane, motion *does* occur in the _____ and _____ planes.

sagittal, frontal

3-3
The axis of the first ray is angulated 45° from *both* the frontal and sagittal planes (Fig. 3.2). Since it is equally angulated from both planes, one might expect the motion available in both the sagittal and frontal planes to be (*equal/unequal*).

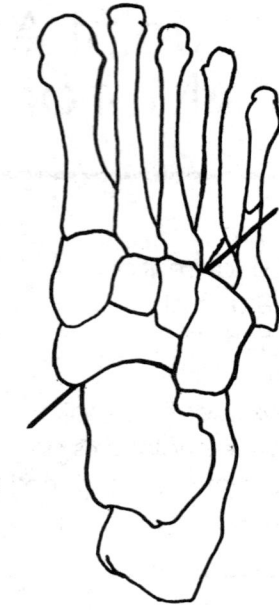

Figure 3.2.
A dorsal view of the first ray's axis. Note its 45° orientation from the sagittal and frontal planes.

equal

3-4
Since the axis of the first ray is angulated equally at 45° from the _____ and _____ planes, the range of clinically observable motion in these two planes is equal. That is, there is as much _____-_____ in the sagittal plane as there is inversion-eversion in the frontal plane.

sagittal, frontal, dorsiflexion, plantarflexion

3-5
So, for every degree of dorsiflexion-plantarflexion in the sagittal plane, there is 1° of _____-_____ in the frontal plane.

inversion, eversion

3-6
Because of the angulation of the axis of the first ray (Fig. 3.3), the dorsiflexion component is coupled with inversion; when plantarflexion occurs, so does eversion. So, when a force (like the ground) pushes the first ray up, it will *simultaneously* dorsiflex and _____.

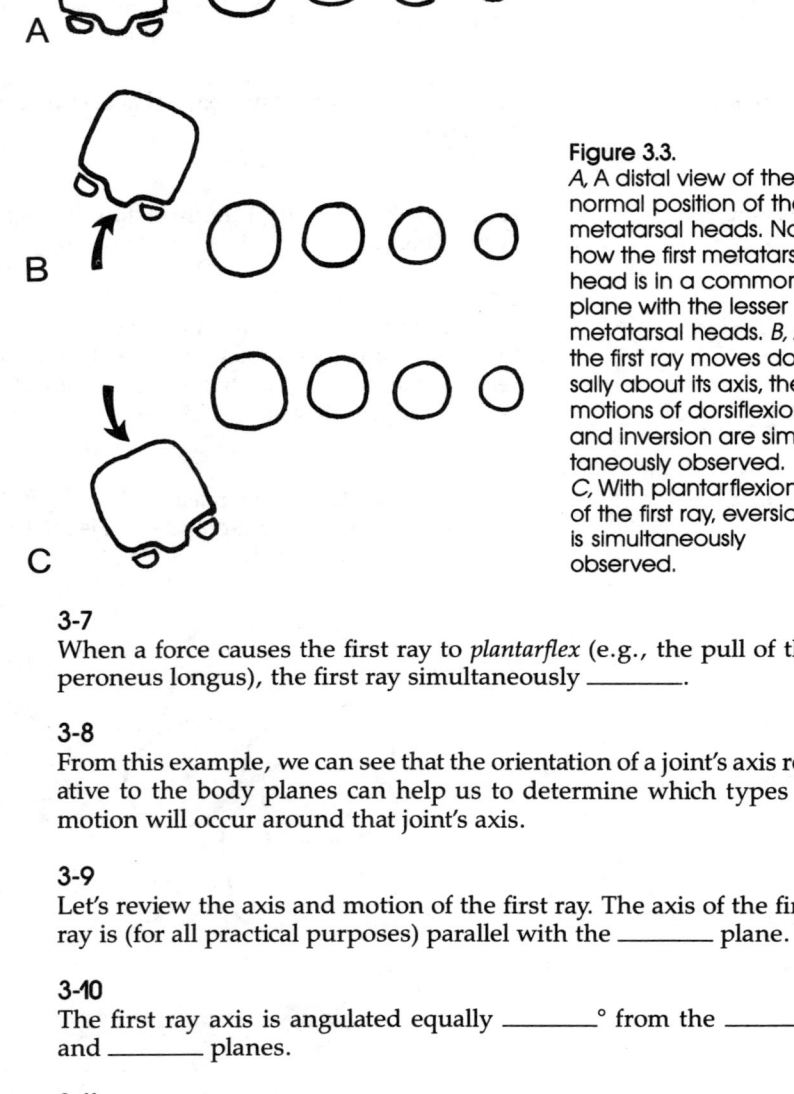

Figure 3.3.
A, A distal view of the normal position of the metatarsal heads. Note how the first metatarsal head is in a common plane with the lesser metatarsal heads. B, As the first ray moves dorsally about its axis, the motions of dorsiflexion and inversion are simultaneously observed. C, With plantarflexion of the first ray, eversion is simultaneously observed.

invert	**3-7** When a force causes the first ray to *plantarflex* (e.g., the pull of the peroneus longus), the first ray simultaneously _____.
everts	**3-8** From this example, we can see that the orientation of a joint's axis relative to the body planes can help us to determine which types of motion will occur around that joint's axis.
	3-9 Let's review the axis and motion of the first ray. The axis of the first ray is (for all practical purposes) parallel with the _____ plane.
transverse	**3-10** The first ray axis is angulated equally _____° from the _____ and _____ planes.
45, sagittal, frontal	**3-11** Since the first ray's axis is equally angulated 45° from the frontal and sagittal planes, the motion which occurs in those planes is *equal/unequal*.
equal	**3-12** That is to say, for every 1° of inversion-eversion that occurs, 1° of _____-_____ occurs.
dorsiflexion, plantarflexion	**3-13** So, first ray motion is equal in the _____ and _____ planes.

sagittal, frontal

3-14
Because of the orientation of the axis from the frontal and sagittal planes, dorsiflexion is coupled with _____ and plantarflexion is coupled with _____.

inversion, eversion

3-15
So, for every 1° of plantarflexion that occurs, 1° of _____ will simultaneously occur.

eversion

3-16
Additionally, for every 1° of inversion that occurs 1° of _____ will occur simultaneously.

dorsiflexion

3-17
Interestingly, the total range of motion (ROM) of the first ray is linked to the position of the subtalar joint (STJ). The motion of the first ray is relatively *increased* when the STJ is *pronated* (that is, when the STJ is everted, abducted, and _____ed).

dorsiflex

3-18
If the first ray's ROM is increased when the STJ is pronated, one may correctly infer that the first ray's ROM is relatively *decreased* when the STJ is in a _____ position (Fig. 3.4).

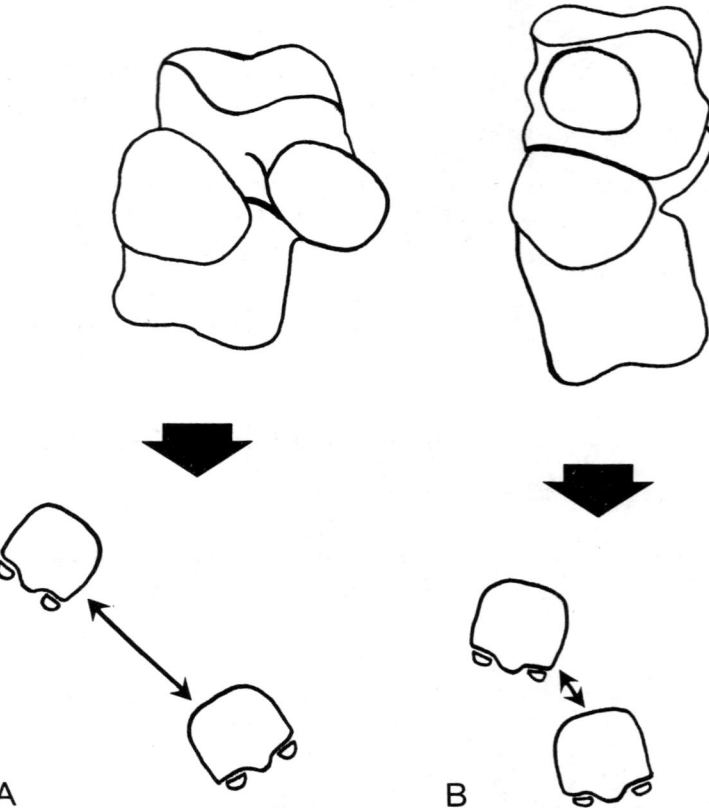

Figure 3.4.
A, A distal view of the subtalar joint (STJ) in a pronated position is at the top. This pronated STJ position will cause the first ray's ROM to be relatively increased. B, When the STJ is in a supinated position, the first ray's RCM is relatively decreased.

3: JOINT AXES AND MOTIONS—FOOT

supinated	**3-19** This follows the general rule that *when the STJ is pronated, the foot becomes a "loose bag of bones."* Conversely, when the foot is supinated, its skeletal structure becomes more rigid. This comes in handy, since the foot must adapt for variance in the terrain (it must be a mobile adaptor), and it must also serve as a *rigid lever* to propel the body forward in space, the latter occurring when the STJ is _____.
supinated	**3-20** While the exact mechanism for the STJ's effect on the first ray is presently unknown, it does seem to follow the rule that *in order for a joint to be stable, the joint(s) proximal to it must be stable.* Since pronation tends to separate the talus and calcaneus (the two bones which compose the STJ), it tends to make the STJ (*more/less*) stable.
less	**3-21** To review, the total ROM of the first ray is affected by the position of the _____.
STJ	**3-22** When the STJ is pronated and therefore relatively (*more/less*) stable, the total ROM of the first ray is relatively (*increased/decreased*).
less, increased	**3-23** This means, therefore, that, in the first ray, more dorsiflexion will occur with _____, and more plantarflexion will occur with _____.
inversion, eversion	**3-24** Since the first ray's axis is practically parallel with the transverse plane (Fig. 3.5), the motion which occurs in that plane is (*great/negligible*), regardless of the STJ's position.

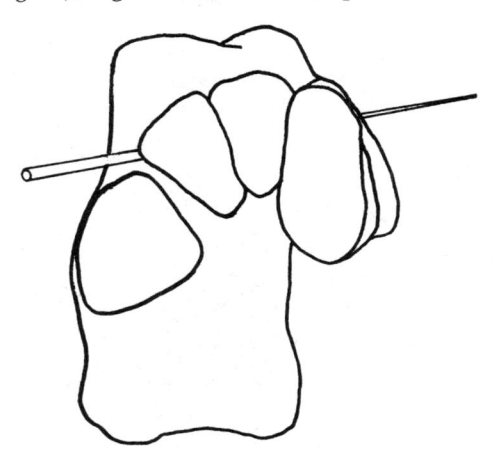

Figure 3.5.
A distal view of the axis of the first ray.

negligible	**3-25** When the foot needs to function as a *rigid lever*, the STJ will be in a relatively _____ position. In this position, the talus and calcaneus are less separated than they are in a _____ position.
supinated, pronated	**3-26** The *most stable* position of the STJ is, therefore, a _____ position.
supinated	**3-27** Since the STJ is relatively *more stable* in a *supinated* position, it will allow the joints distal to it to be (*more/less*) stable as well. (We will go further into STJ function in Chapters 5 and 6).
more	**3-28** Since the STJ has triplane motion (i.e., pronation and supination), one may assume that its axis is (*parallel with/not parallel with*) the three body planes.
not parallel with	**3-29** This is because the only time that motion can*not* occur in a given plane is when the joint axis is parallel with that plane. An example of this would be the first ray's lack of motion in the _____ plane, since its axis is parallel with that plane.
transverse	**3-30** Since the STJ axis (Fig. 3.6) is not parallel with any of the three body planes, it has motion occurring in all three body planes. These two triplane motions are called _____ and _____.

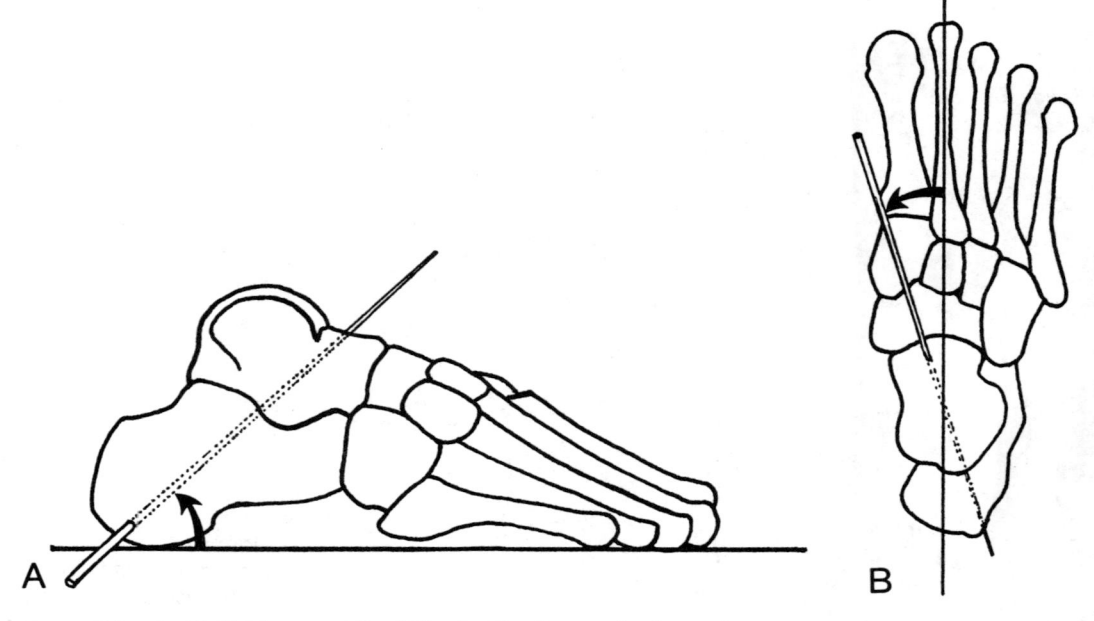

Figure 3.6. *A*, A lateral view of the STJ axis. (The line under the calcaneus and metatarsals represents the transverse plane.) *B*, A dorsal view of the STJ axis. (The line running through the second metatarsal represents the sagittal plane as it passes through the midline of the foot.)

3: JOINT AXES AND MOTIONS—FOOT

pronation, supination

3-31
Pronation is a triplane motion consisting of simultaneous movements of abduction, dorsiflexion, and eversion. Supination is a triplane motion which combines the movements of adduction, _____ and _____ (Fig. 3.7).

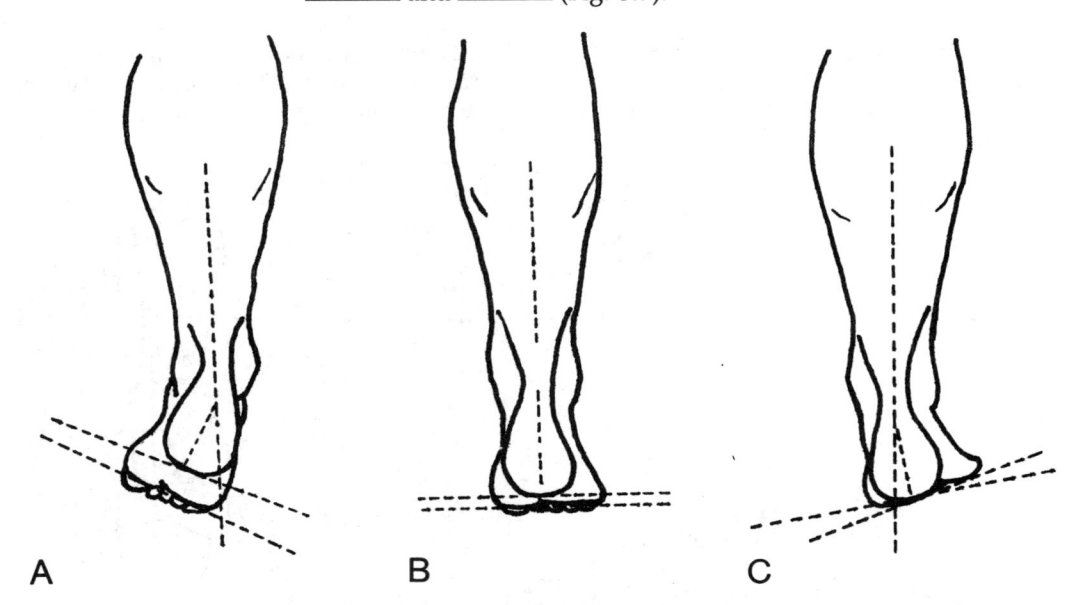

Figure 3.7. *A,* The STJ and foot in a supinated position. *B,* The STJ and foot in their neutral positions. *C,* The STJ and foot in a pronated position.

plantarflexion, inversion

3-32
The STJ axis, around which this motion occurs, runs from *distal, medial,* and *dorsal* (pneumonic = D.M.D.) to *proximal, plantar,* and *lateral* (Fig. 3.8).

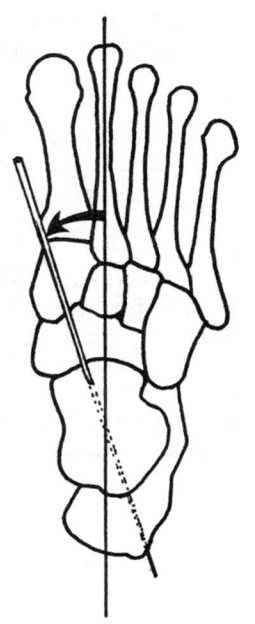

Figure 3.8.
A dorsal view of the STJ axis.

3-33
To describe the spatial orientation of the STJ axis, one would say that it runs from proximal, lateral, and plantar to _____, _____, and _____ (HINT: dentist's degree).

distal, medial, dorsal

3-34
(Fig. 3.9) Specifically, the STJ axis is angulated 16° from the sagittal plane and 42° from the transverse plane. This specific orientation must be memorized: Sixteen from Sagittal and forty-Two from Transverse.

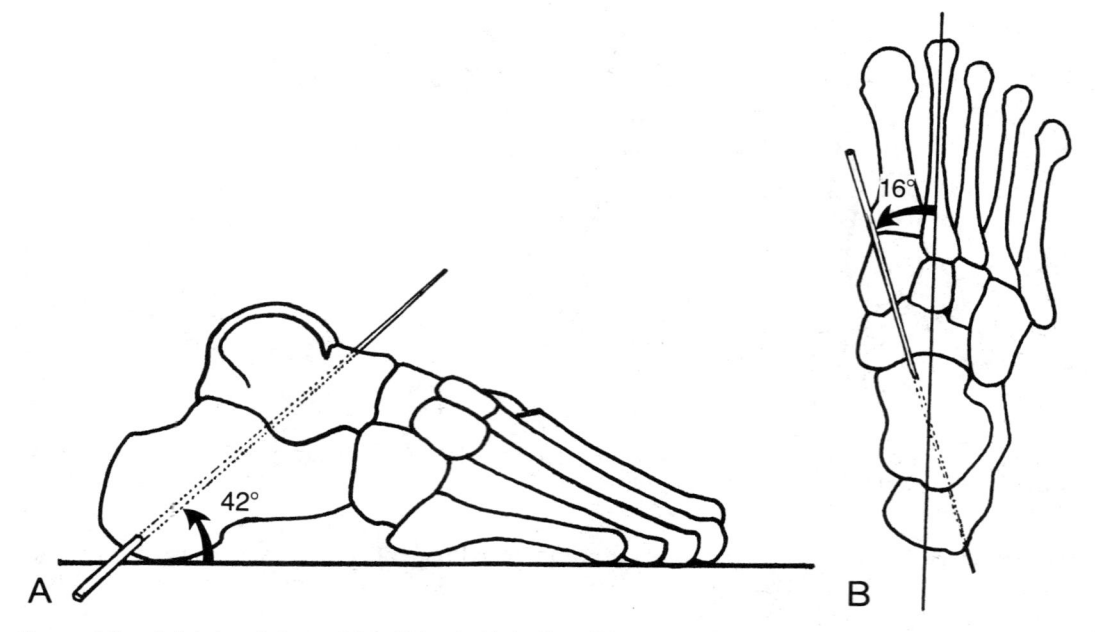

Figure 3.9. A, A lateral view of the STJ axis. Note the 42° angulation from the transverse plane. B, A dorsal view of the STJ axis. Note the 16° angulation from the sagittal plane.

3-35
So, the STJ axis, which runs from proximal, lateral, and plantar to _____, _____, and _____ is angulated Sixteen degrees from the _____ plane and forty-Two degrees from the _____ plane.

distal, medial, dorsal,
Sagittal, Transverse

3-36
To summarize, pronation and supination of the STJ occur about an axis that is angulated _____° from the _____ plane and _____° from the _____ plane.

16, sagittal
42, transverse

3-37
The STJ axis runs from _____, _____, and _____ to _____, _____, and _____.

3: JOINT AXES AND MOTIONS—FOOT

3-38

distal, medial, dorsal, (to) proximal, plantar, lateral

(Fig. 3.10) The axis of the first ray is somewhat opposite of the STJ in the way it runs. While the STJ axis runs from *distal, medial,* and dorsal to *proximal, lateral,* and plantar, the *first ray axis* runs from *distal-lateral* to *proximal-medial.*

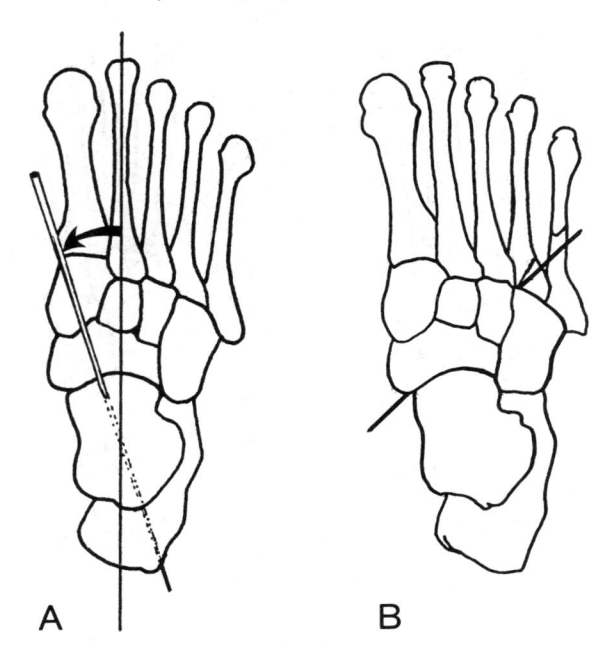

Figure 3.10.
A, A dorsal view of the STJ axis. *B,* A dorsal view of the first ray axis.

3-39

We don't worry about the dorsal-plantar relation to the first ray's axis since it lies parallel with the _____ plane.

3-40

transverse

The first ray's axis runs somewhat opposite of the STJ's axis in that the first ray's axis runs from distal-_____ to proximal-_____ and is angulated equally _____° from both the sagittal and frontal planes.

3-41

lateral, medial, 45

It is interesting to note that the fifth ray's axis runs in the same spatial orientation as the STJ's axis, which is from _____, _____, and _____ to _____, _____, and _____ (Fig. 3.11).

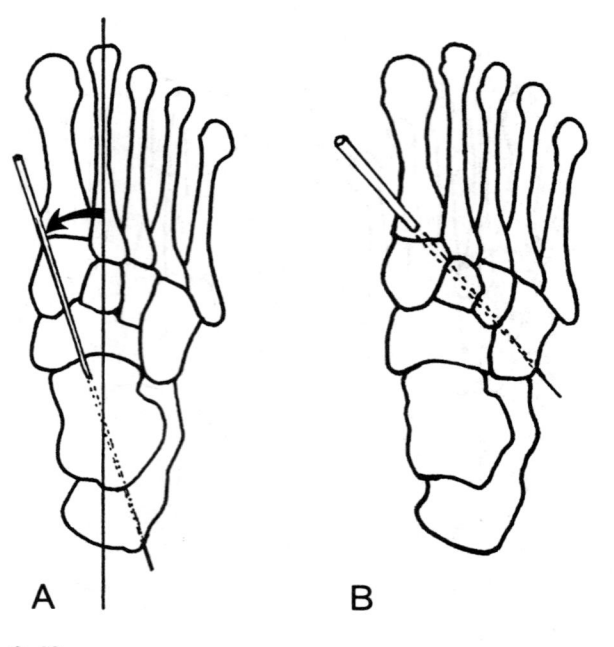

Figure 3.11.
A, A dorsal view of the STJ axis. B, A dorsal view of the fifth ray axis.

3-42

distal, medial, dorsal to proximal, plantar, lateral

Since the fifth ray's axis runs in the same spatial orientation (roughly) as does the STJ's axis, one may correctly assume that the fifth ray's axis is also a (*monoplane/biplane/triplane*) axis.

3-43

triplane

This is true, as you recall from the previous chapter, that an axis which is angulated with all three body planes is called a _____ axis.

3-44

triplane

Since this type of axis does not rest parallel with any one body plane, motion occurs in all three planes. An example of how a joint axis can rest parallel with one body plane and therefore not allow motion in that one plane would be found in the axis of the _____ ray.

3: JOINT AXES AND MOTIONS—FOOT

first

3-45
In the first ray, the axis is parallel with the _____ plane and equally angulated _____° from the _____ and _____ planes (Fig. 3.12).

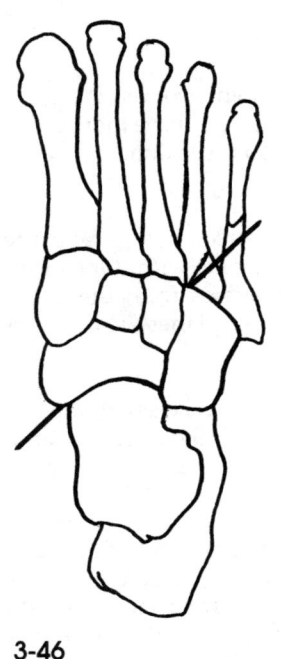

Figure 3.12.
A dorsal view of the first ray axis.

transverse, 45, sagittal, frontal

3-46
So, to review, the axes of the _____ ray and _____ joint run in the same spatial orientation going from distal, medial, and dorsal to proximal, lateral, and plantar.

fifth, subtalar

3-47
The axis of the first ray runs somewhat opposite this orientation by running from _____-_____ to _____-_____.

distal-lateral, proximal-medial

3-48
Since pronation and supination occur about the triplane axis of the STJ, one may correctly infer that the same motions take place about the triplane axis of the _____ ray.

fifth

3-49
While the axes of the STJ and fifth ray share roughly the same spatial orientation, there are other joints in the foot which share a different spatial orientation. These are the *interphalangeal joints (IPJs)*, the *metatarsophalangeal joints (MPJs)*, and the *central three rays*.

3-50
The central three rays, along with the _____ and IPJs, have axes that are parallel (for practical purposes) with the *frontal* and *transverse* planes.

MPJs

3-51
Since the central three rays, as well as the MPJs and IPJs have axes parallel with the _____ and _____ planes, it is reasonable to assume that all of these joints will have motion *only* in the _____ plane.

frontal, transverse, sagittal

3-52
In fact, all of these joint groups (the _____ _____ _____, the _____ and the _____ have motion only in the sagittal plane, i.e., dorsiflexion and plantarflexion.

central three rays, MPJs, IPJs

3-53
This makes sense, since the sagittal plane is the only plane that the joint axes are *not* parallel with. One of these joint groups, however, has another *separate* axis from the one which is parallel with the frontal and transverse planes. This group is the MPJs.

3-54
Three joint groups share axes with the same spatial orientation—the _____ _____ rays, the _____, and the _____. Only one of these groups, the _____, has a separate axis.

central three, MPJs, IPJs, MPJs

3-55
In addition to the axis parallel with the *frontal and transverse* planes, the MPJs have a separate axis which is parallel with the *frontal and sagittal* planes. These two axes of the MPJs can be classified respectively as the *horizontal axis* and the *vertical axis* (Fig. 3.13).

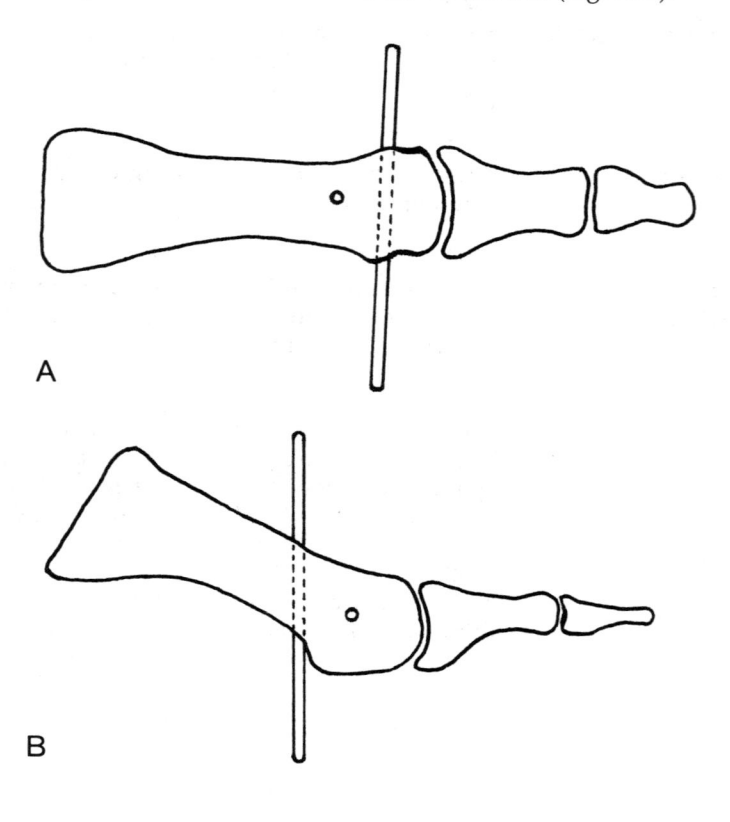

Figure 3.13.
A, A dorsal view of the axes of the MPJ. *B*, A lateral view of the axes of the MPJ.

3: JOINT AXES AND MOTIONS—FOOT 33

3-56
So, out of the central three rays, the IPJs, and the MPJs, only the _____ have two separate axes—a horizontal one which is parallel with the frontal and transverse planes and a vertical one which is parallel with the frontal and sagittal planes.

MPJs

3-57
We know that joint groups which have axes parallel with the frontal and transverse planes only have motion available in the _____ plane. Regarding the MPJs' vertical axis, which is parallel with the frontal and sagittal planes, one would expect there to be motion only in the _____ plane.

sagittal, transverse

3-58
This is true since motion can only occur in a plane if the joint axis (*is/is not*) parallel with that plane.

is not

3-59
So, the MPJs have dorsiflexion-plantarflexion motion about their _____ axis and the motions of abduction-adduction about their _____ axis.

horizontal, vertical

3-60
The three groups of joints which have sagittal plane motion around their axes which are parallel to the frontal and _____ planes are the _____ _____ _____, the _____, and the _____.

transverse, central three rays, MPJs, IPJs

3-61
To review, we know that the first ray's axis is parallel with the _____ plane and is angulated equally _____° from the _____ and _____ planes.

transverse, 45, frontal, sagittal

3-62
Because of the spatial orientation of the first ray axis (somewhat opposite the STJ and fifth ray axes) running from _____-_____ to _____-_____, dorsiflexion occurs with equal amounts of _____ and plantarflexion occurs with equal amounts of _____.

distal-lateral, proximal-medial, inversion, eversion

3-63
As mentioned above, the STJ and fifth ray have axes which run somewhat opposite of the first ray axis. That is, the axes for the STJ and fifth ray run from _____, _____, and _____ to _____, _____, and _____.

distal, medial, dorsal, proximal, lateral, plantar

3-64
Since these are (*monoplane/biplane/triplane*) axes, the motion which occurs around them is _____ motion.

triplane, triplane

3-65
This motion is called _____ and supination.

pronation

3-66
The STJ axis is angulated _____° from the sagittal plane and _____° from the transverse plane.

34   FOOT FUNCTION: A PROGRAMMED TEXT

16, 42

3-67
The three joint groups which have axes that are parallel to the frontal and transverse planes are the _____ _____ _____, the _____, and the _____.

central three rays, IPJs, MPJs

3-68
These joint groups exhibit motion in what plane about their axes?

sagittal

3-69
The joint group which has a separate axis in addition to the one identified above is the _____.

MPJs

3-70
The MPJs have two axes: a vertical one which is parallel to the _____ and _____ planes and a horizontal one which is parallel to the _____ and _____ planes.

frontal, sagittal, frontal, transverse

3-71
The motions which occur about the horizontal axis are _____ and _____. The motions occurring about the vertical axis are _____ and _____.

dorsiflexion, plantarflexion, abduction, adduction

3-72
You're doing very well! We just have one more joint to examine—the *midtarsal joint (MTJ)*. The MTJ also has two separate axes, just like the _____.

MPJs

3-73
The MTJ has two axes: a *longitudinal* axis and an *oblique* axis (Fig. 3.14).

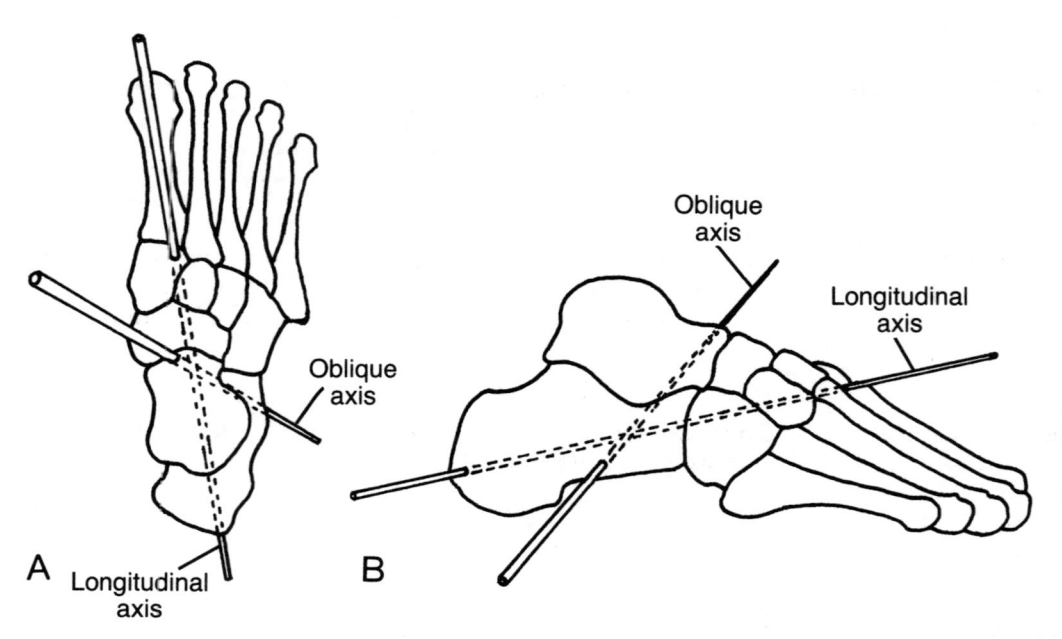

Figure 3.14. *A*, A dorsal view of the MTJ axes. *B*, A lateral view of the MTJ axes.

3: JOINT AXES AND MOTIONS—FOOT

Although, in reality, triplane motion occurs about both MTJ axes, some planes of motion are so small as to be clinically insignificant.

Triplane motion about the axes of the MTJ is important in purely academic circles. However, *for the practical purposes of this book*, we will talk about there being only one or two planes of motion about a particular MTJ axis.

3-74
Just like the MPJs, the MTJ has (*one/two/three*) axis/axes.

3-75
two

The two MTJ axes are called the longitudinal and _____ axes.

3-76
oblique

The longitudinal axis is just about parallel with the transverse and sagittal planes. Therefore (for practical purposes), motion will only occur in the _____ plane.

3-77
frontal

The MTJ axis, which is parallel with the transverse and sagittal planes, is called the _____ axis and allows motion only in the frontal plane—i.e., inversion and _____.

3-78
longitudinal, eversion

The MTJ longitudinal axis is parallel with the _____ and _____ planes and allows only the motions of _____ and _____ to occur about it.

3-79
transverse, sagittal, inversion, eversion

The MTJ longitudinal axis allows motion only in the _____ plane, since it is parallel with the _____ and _____ planes.

frontal, transverse, sagittal

3-80
The other MTJ axis, the _____ axis, is almost parallel with the frontal plane. Because of this spatial orientation, it allows motion in both the transverse and sagittal planes (Fig. 3.15).

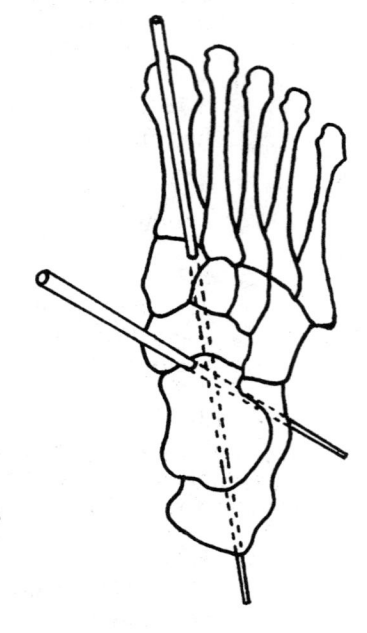

Figure 3.15.
A dorsal view of the MTJ axes. Note how the MTJ oblique axis is almost parallel to a frontal plane.

oblique

3-81
So, the MTJ longitudinal axis allows motion in the _____ plane, while the MTJ oblique axis allows motion in the _____ and _____ planes.

frontal, transverse, sagittal

3-82
The MTJ oblique axis motion is coupled so that when there is dorsiflexion there is also abduction. Conversely, when there is plantarflexion, there is also _____.

adduction

3-83
So, to review the MTJ, we can say that it has (*one/two/three*) axis/axes.

3: JOINT AXES AND MOTIONS—FOOT   37

two

3-84
These two axes are called the _____ and _____ axes of the MTJ (Fig. 3.16).

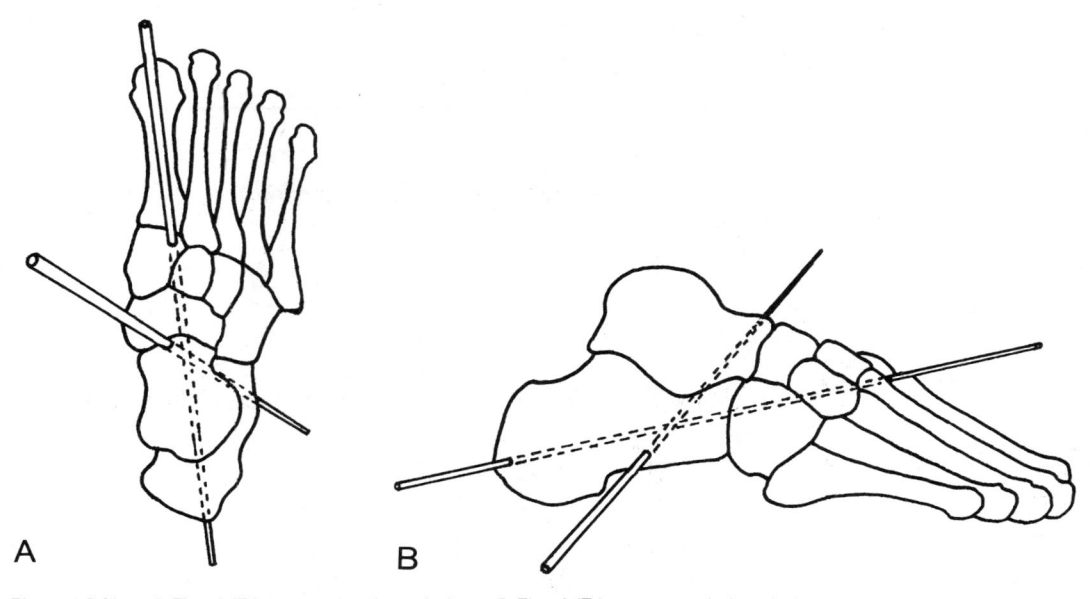

Figure 3.16. A, The MTJ axes—a dorsal view. B, The MTJ axes—a lateral view.

longitudinal, oblique

3-85
The longitudinal axis is essentially parallel with which two planes?

transverse, sagittal

3-86
Since the longitudinal axis is parallel with the transverse and sagittal planes, the only motion it allows is _____ plane motion, i.e., _____ and _____.

frontal, inversion, eversion

3-87
The MTJ oblique axis is essentially parallel with the _____ plane. The only motion that it allows is in the _____ and _____ planes.

frontal, transverse, sagittal

3-88
The motion about the MTJ oblique axis consists of two coupled motions: 1) _____ with _____ and 2) _____ with _____.

dorsiflexion, abduction, plantarflexion, adduction

3-89
This completes the chapter on axes and motion of the joints of the foot. If you need a quick review, you can read over frames 3-60 through 3-70 and frames 3-83 through 3-88.

Questions

FRAME 3-3

1. The first ray is equally angulated 45° from the:
   a. sagittal plane
   b. frontal plane
   c. transverse plane
   d. a and b
   e. a and c

FRAME 3-6

2. With regard to first ray motion, dorsiflexion is clinically coupled with an equal amount of:
   a. adduction
   b. abduction
   c. inversion
   d. eversion
   e. supination

FRAME 3-19

3. STJ supination will decrease the first ray's ROM.
   a. true
   b. false

FRAME 3-34

4. An axis which is angulated 42° from the transverse plane and 16° from the sagittal plane describes the:
   a. metatarsophalangeal joint axis
   b. MTJ longitudinal axis
   c. MTJ oblique axis
   d. STJ axis
   e. ankle joint axis

FRAME 3-32

5. The STJ axis runs from _____, _____, and _____ to _____, _____, and _____.
   a. distal, lateral, dorsal to proximal, medial, plantar
   b. distal, lateral, plantar to proximal, medial, dorsal
   c. distal, medial, plantar to proximal, lateral, dorsal
   d. distal, medial, dorsal to proximal, lateral, plantar
   e. none of the above

FRAME 3-49

6. Axes that are (for practical purposes) parallel with the frontal and transverse planes describe an axis of the:
   a. IPJs
   b. MPJs
   c. central three rays
   d. a and b
   e. a, b, and c

3: JOINT AXES AND MOTIONS—FOOT

FRAME 3-55

7. The MTJ is the only joint in the foot that has two axes.
    a. true
    b. false

FRAMES 3-56—3-59

8. The MPJ allows motion to occur about its axes in which plane(s)?
    a. sagittal
    b. frontal
    c. transverse
    d. a and b
    e. a and c

FRAMES 3-75—3-77

9. The MTJ longitudinal axis allows motion primarily in which plane(s)?
    a. sagittal
    b. frontal
    c. transverse
    d. a and b
    e. a and c

FRAME 3-82

10. With dorsiflexion about the MTJ oblique axis, there must also be:
    a. adduction
    b. abduction
    c. inversion
    d. eversion
    e. supination

Answers

1. d	4. d	7. b	10. b
2. c	5. d	8. e	
3. a	6. e	9. b	

CHAPTER 4

Overview of the Gait Cycle

- gait cycle definition
- stance phase
- swing phase
- periods of the stance phase
- foot function during the gait cycle

4-1
The gait cycle is defined as that interval of time from heel strike of one foot to heel strike by the same foot at the next step. The events that take place within this period are divided into two major components: the *stance phase* and the *swing phase* of gait (Fig. 4.1).

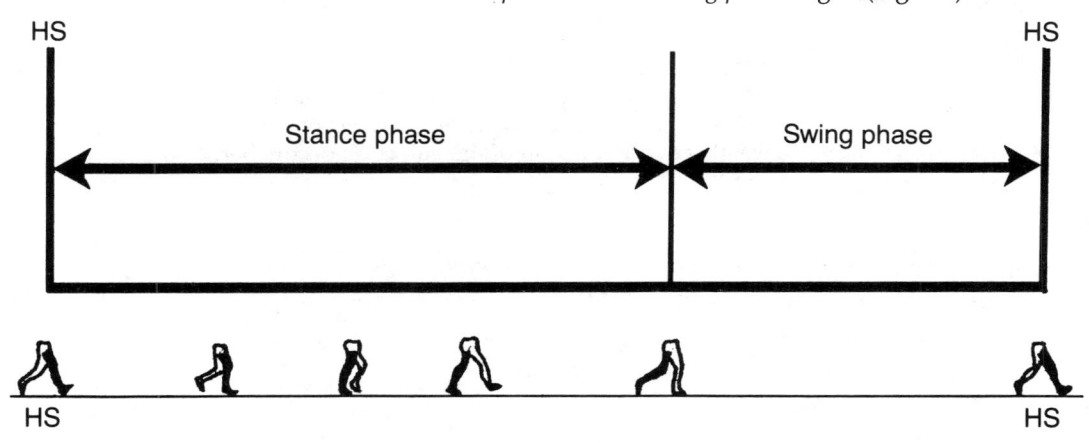

Figure 4.1. The gait cycle occurs between heel strike (HS) of one foot and that foot's next HS.

4-2
The two major components of the gait cycle, the _____ phase and the _____ phase, occur between heel strike of one foot and the next heel strike of that same foot.

stance, swing

4-3
As you may infer, the stance phase occurs during the weightbearing period of the gait cycle while the swing phase occurs during the non-weightbearing portion of the gait cycle.

4-4
Besides *heel strike*, other significant hallmarks of the gait cycle include *forefoot loading, heel lift,* and *toe off* (Fig. 4.2). The non-weightbearing portion of the gait cycle, i.e., the _____ phase, occurs between toe off and heel strike of the same foot.

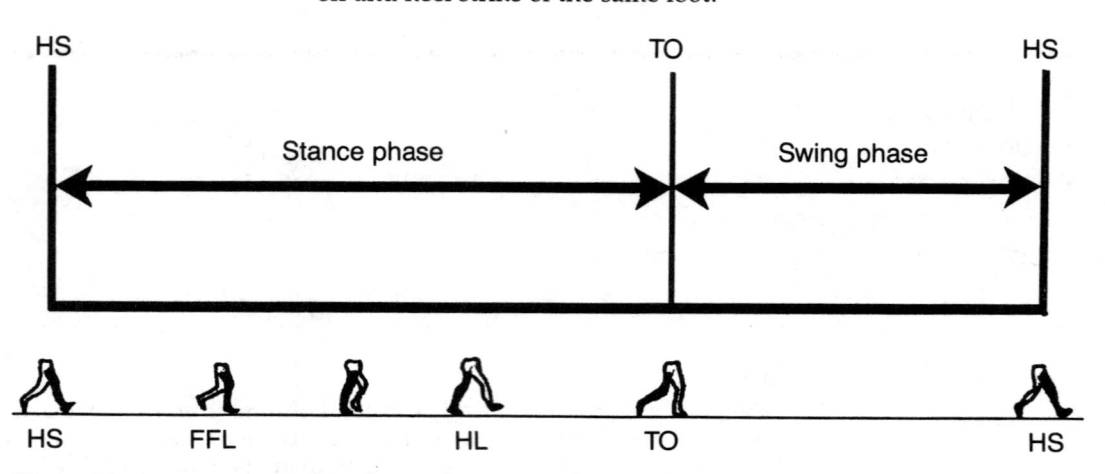

Figure 4.2. Hallmarks of the gait cycle include heel strike (HS), forefoot loading (FFL), heel lift (HL), and toe off (TO).

swing

4-5
The weightbearing portion of the gait cycle, i.e., the _____ phase, occurs between heel strike and toe off of the same foot. The non-weightbearing portion of the gait cycle occurs between _____ and _____.

stance, toe off, heel strike

4-6
The stance phase occupies a majority of the gait cycle—approximately 60%. The swing phase occupies the remainder of the cycle, about 40% (Fig. 4.3).

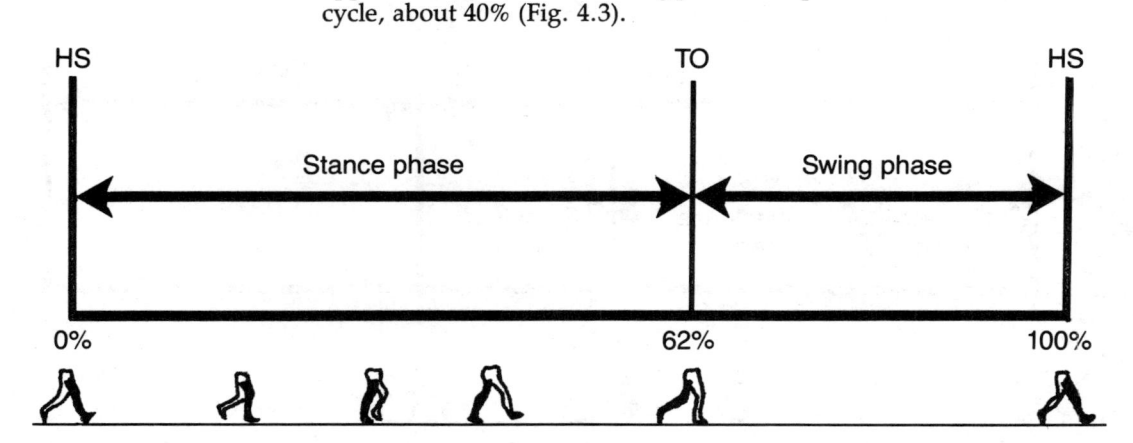

Figure 4.3. The stance phase of gait occupies 62% of the gait cycle while the swing phase occupies only 38% of the gait cycle. For our purposes, we will round these off to 60% and 40% respectively.

4-7
During the swing phase, which occupies about _____% of the gait cycle, the foot pronates first and then supinates.

4-8
Pronation shortens the foot, which helps it to clear the ground. Pronation also minimizes the energy expenditure necessary for ground clearance as the non-weightbearing limb passes the weightbearing limb. Supination stabilizes the bony architecture of the foot thus preparing it for heel strike.

4-9
The stance phase occupies about _____% of the gait cycle.

60

4-10

The stance phase is divided into three named periods. In order of occurrence (as well as alphabetical order), they are the *contact period*, the *midstance period*, and the *propulsive period* (Fig. 4.4).

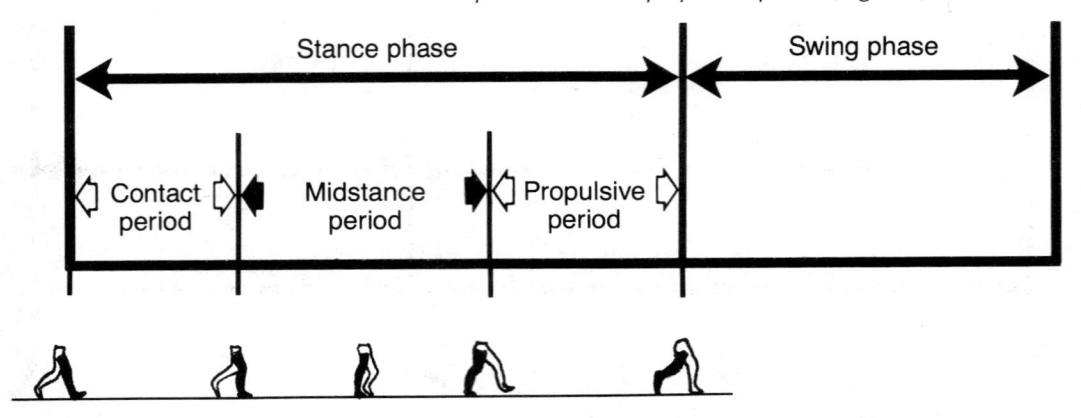

Figure 4.4. The contact, midstance, and propulsive periods compose the stance phase of the gait cylce.

4-11

The three periods of the stance phase of gait, in the order of their occurrence, are the _____, _____, and _____ periods.

contact, midstance, propulsive

4-12

The contact, midstance, and propulsive periods respectively take up about *30%, 40%,* and *30%* of the stance phase of gait (Fig. 4.5). The stance phase of gait occupies about _____ % of the total gait cycle.

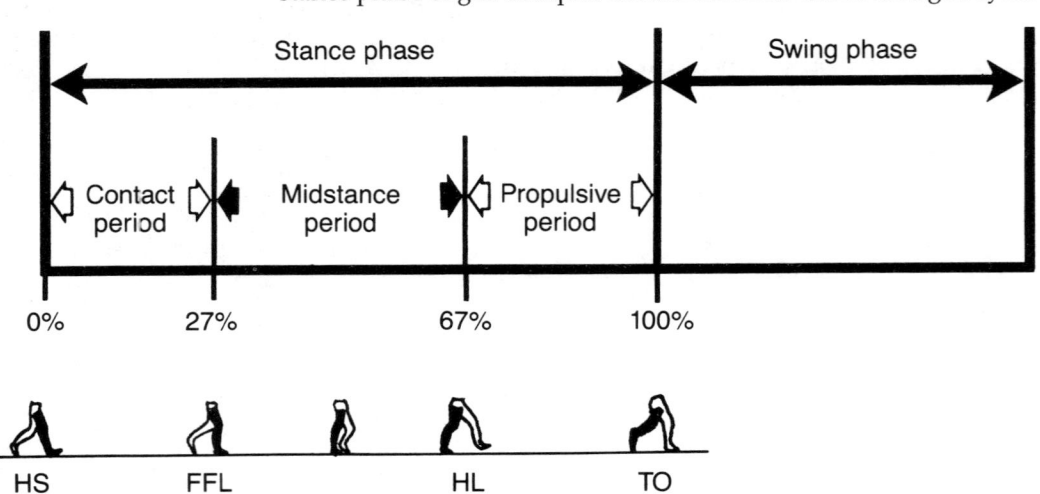

Figure 4.5. The contact period occupies 27% of the stance phase of the gait cycle; the midstance perioc, 40%; the propulsive period, 33%. We round these off to 30%, 40%, and 30%, respectively.

4: OVERVIEW OF THE GAIT CYCLE

60

4-13
The midstance period of the _____ phase of gait occupies about _____ % of that phase.

stance, 40

4-14
Both the contact and propulsive periods each take up _____ % of the stance phase of gait.

30

4-15
The stance phase of gait occurs between heel strike and _____ _____ of the same foot. The contact period occurs between heel strike of the same foot and toe off of the opposite foot (Fig. 4.6). Note that forefoot loading occurs in the foot that is finishing its contact period at the same time that toe off is occurring in the opposite foot.

So, the contact period of the right foot occurs between heel strike of the (*right/left*) foot and toe off of the (*right/left*) foot.

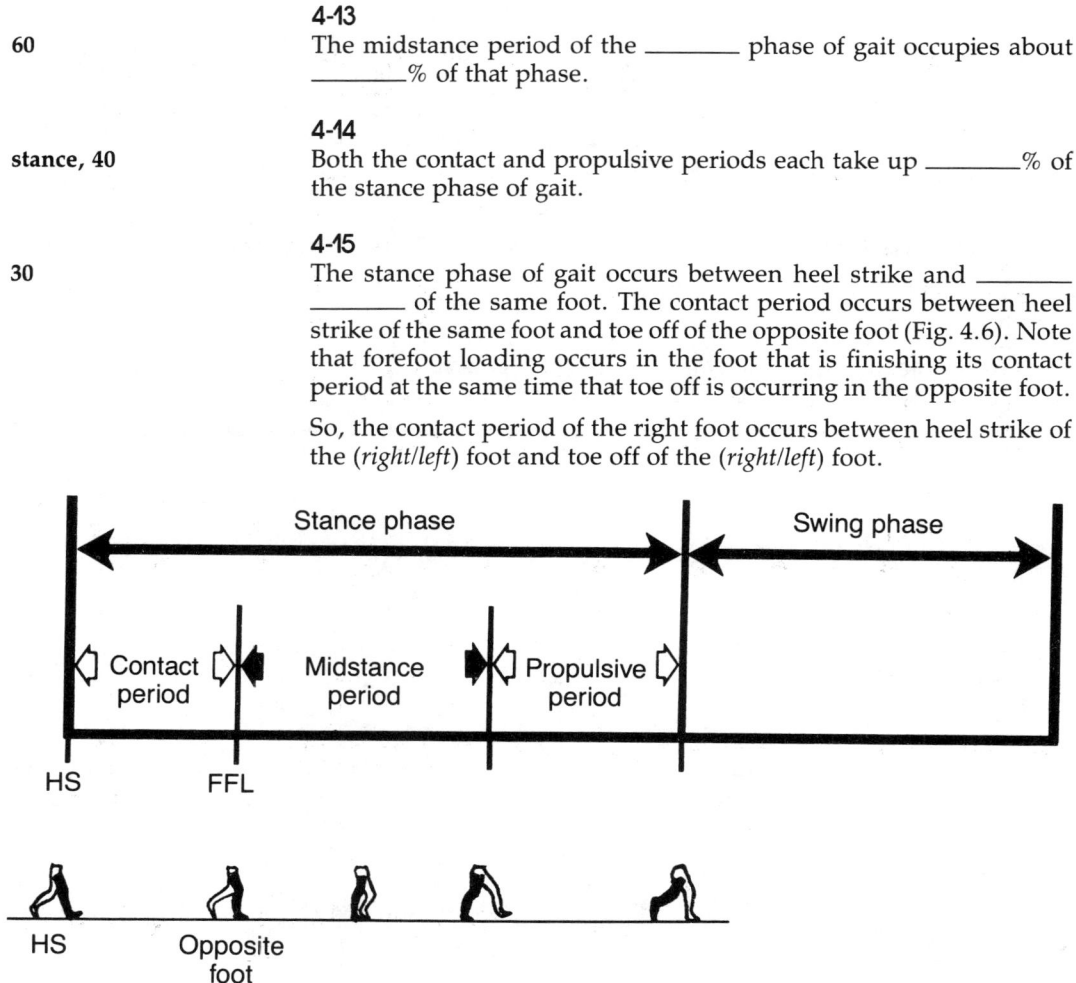

Figure 4.6. The contact period occupies roughly the first 30% of the stance period. Forefoot loading (FFL) occurs as the contact period ends and the midstance period begins.

toe off, right, left

4-16
The period directly following the contact period is the _____ period.

midstance

4-17
The midstance period starts just after the end of the contact period, i.e., right after toe off of the (*same/opposite*) foot.

opposite

4-18
So, the period of the stance phase of gait which goes from heel strike of the same foot to toe off of the opposite foot is the _____ period.

contact

4-19
The midstance period starts just after _____ _____ of the opposite foot and ends with heel lift of the same foot.

46   FOOT FUNCTION: A PROGRAMMED TEXT

toe off

4-20
Heel lift not only ends the midstance period of the stance phase of gait, but it also begins the propulsive period (Fig. 4.7). The propulsive period is the last part of the stance phase to occur, thus it ends with the same thing that ends the stance phase—_____ _____ of the same foot.

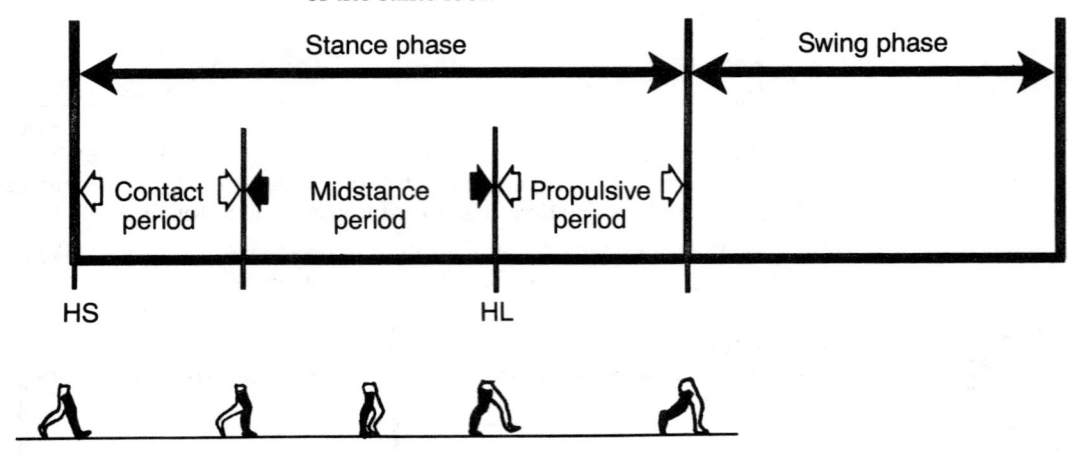

Figure 4.7. Heel lift (HL) signifies both the end of the midstance period and the beginning of the propulsive period.

toe off

4-21
The stance phase of gait is divided into three periods which follow each other. In order, they are the _____, _____, and _____ periods of stance phase.

contact, midstance, propulsive

4-22
The period between heel lift and toe off of the same foot is the _____ period.

propulsive

4-23
The period between toe off of the opposite foot and heel lift of the same foot is the _____ period.

midstance

4-24
The phase of gait which occurs between toe off of one foot and heel strike of the same foot is the _____ phase of gait.

swing

4-25
The period which occurs between heel strike of one foot and toe off of the opposite foot is the _____ period of gait.

contact

4-26
During the swing phase, the foot first (*pronates/supinates*) and then (*pronates/supinates*) (Fig. 4.8).

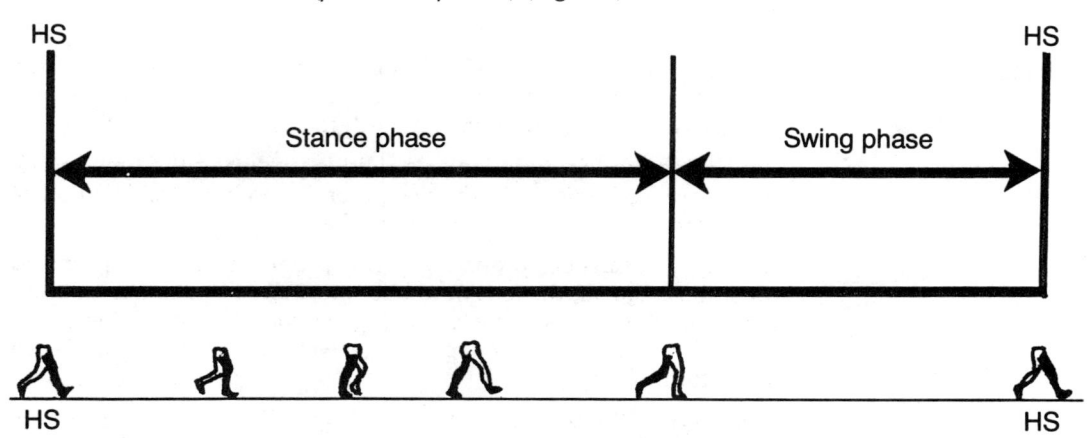

Figure 4.8. The gait cycle occurs between heel strike (HS) of one foot and that foot's next HS.

pronates, supinates

4-27
At the beginning of weightbearing, during the entire contact period, the STJ pronates in order to make the foot more flexible and, as such, a better mobile adaptor to variances in terrain.

4-28
After the contact period, during which the STJ (*pronates/supinates*), the STJ supinates until just before the end of the propulsive period (Fig. 4.9).

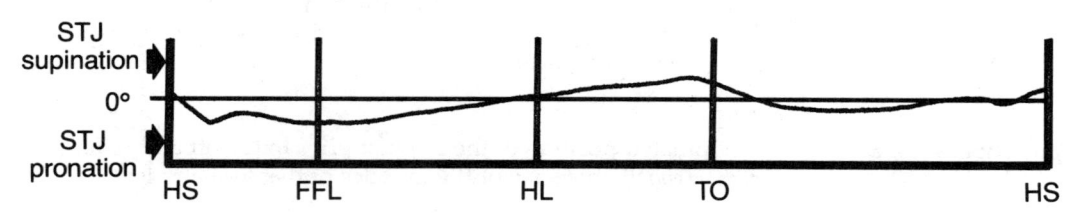

Figure 4.9. STJ motion during the gait cycle.

pronates	**4-29** So, during the midstance and most of the propulsive periods, the STJ is (*pronating/supinating*).
supinating	**4-30** Through supinating the STJ during the midstance and most of the propulsive periods, the foot is converted from a mobile adaptor (which it is during the contact period) to a rigid lever. By having the foot function as a rigid lever during the time immediately preceding toe off, the weight of the body is propelled off of that limb with the greatest mechanical efficiency. If the STJ was instead pronating during propulsion and in a pronated position at toe off, the foot would become more of a _____ adaptor and, therefore, a relatively "loose bag of bones." It would, therefore, take more muscle energy to propel the weight of the body off of such a platform. Some types of foot pathology cause abnormal pronation during propulsion and a pronated position at the end of propulsion. As a result, there is significant foot and leg fatigue secondary to overuse of muscles. Additionally, abnormal pronation during the propulsive period causes *hypermobility* (an unstable state of joints which are supposed to be stable) and *abnormal shearing forces* between the bones and skin of the forefoot. The latter produces skin calluses, while the former causes joint subluxations. (More on this in Chapter 11.)
mobile	**4-31** So, during the contact period, the foot is a mobile adaptor because of STJ (*pronation/supination*). During the midstance and most of the propulsive periods, the foot becomes a rigid lever secondary to progressive (*pronation/supination*) of the STJ.
pronation, supination	**4-32** A supinated position of the STJ just prior to toe off allows for (*minimal/maximal*) efficiency of the muscles of that foot and leg.
maximal	**4-33** Fatigue of the muscles of the foot and leg can result from a (*supinated/pronated*) position of the STJ just prior to toe off.
pronated	**4-34** This completes the overview of the gait cycle. More specific information will be covered in further chapters regarding normal and pathological joint motion during the gait cycle.

Questions

FRAME 4-4

1. The portion of the gait cycle which occurs between toe off and heel strike of the same foot is called the:

   a. contact period
   b. midstance period
   c. propulsive period
   d. stance phase
   e. swing phase

FRAME 4-7

2. During the swing phase, the foot supinates first and then pronates.

   a. true
   b. false

FRAMES 4-17 AND 4-19

3. Which portion of the gait cycle occurs between toe off of the opposite foot and heel lift of the same foot.

   a. contact period
   b. midstance period
   c. propulsive period
   d. stance phase
   e. swing phase

FRAME 4-15

4. Which part of the gait cycle occurs between heel strike of the same foot and toe off of the opposite foot?

   a. contact period
   b. midstance period
   c. propulsive period
   d. stance phase
   e. swing phase

FRAME 4-10

5. The order of the periods of the stance phase, from beginning to end, is:

   a. propulsive, contact, midstance
   b. propulsive, midstance, contact
   c. contact, midstance, propulsive
   d. contact, propulsive, midstance
   e. midstance, contact, propulsive

FRAME 4-27

6. During the entire contact period of gait, the STJ pronates.

   a. true
   b. false

FRAME 4-30

7. The foot is converted from a mobile adaptor into a rigid lever during which part of the gait cycle?
   a. contact period
   b. midstance period
   c. propulsive period
   d. stance phase
   e. swing phase

FRAME 4-30

8. It is important that the STJ be supinating during the propulsive period of gait in order to let the foot function as a rigid lever.
   a. true
   b. false

FRAME 4-27

9. The foot functions most as mobile adaptor during which part of the gait cylce?
   a. contact period
   b. midstance period
   c. propulsive period
   d. stance phase
   e. swing phase

FRAMES 4-30 AND 4-33

10. Fatigue of the muscles of the foot and leg can most result from a pronated position of the STJ just prior to:
    a. heel strike
    b. stance phase
    c. forefoot loading
    d. midstance period
    e. toe off

Answers

1. e
2. b
3. b
4. a
5. c
6. a
7. b
8. a
9. a
10. e

CHAPTER 5

Subtalar Joint Function in Open and Closed Kinetic Chain

- open and closed kinetic chain definition
- STJ component motions in open and closed kinetic chain
- tibial rotations related to STJ motions
- STJ motions during the stance phase
- STJ motions during the swing phase

5-1
Open and closed kinetic chain respectively refer to states of non-weightbearing and weightbearing. So, if the right lower limb is bearing weight, it is said to be functioning in (*open/closed*) kinetic chain.

closed

5-2
Conversely, if a right lower limb is functioning in open kinetic chain, it (*is/is not*) weightbearing.

is not

5-3
A joint may exhibit different component motions in open versus closed kinetic chain function. Such is the case with the STJ.

5-4
Recall that during the gait cycle, the STJ functions during both the weightbearing and non-weightbearing portions. During the first half of the swing phase, the STJ (*pronates/supinates*). During the last half of the swing phase, the STJ (*pronates/supinates*) (Fig. 5.1). The swing phase is (*open/closed*) kinetic chain.

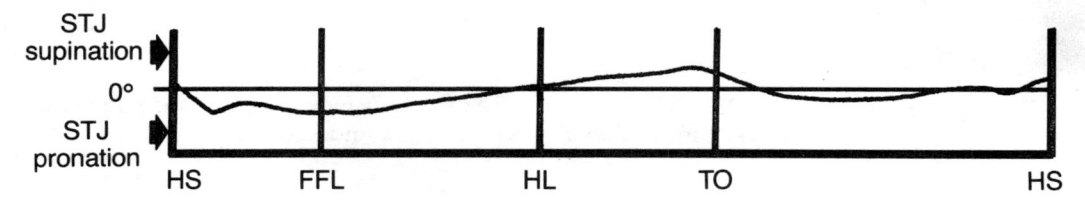

Figure 5.1. STJ motion during the gait cycle.

pronates, supinates, open

5-5
In open kinetic chain (OKC) function, the STJ pronatory and supinatory components are exhibited exclusively by the calcaneus (Fig. 5.2). That is to say with *OKC pronation*, the calcaneus abducts, everts, and (*dorsiflexes/plantarflexes*).

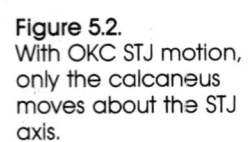

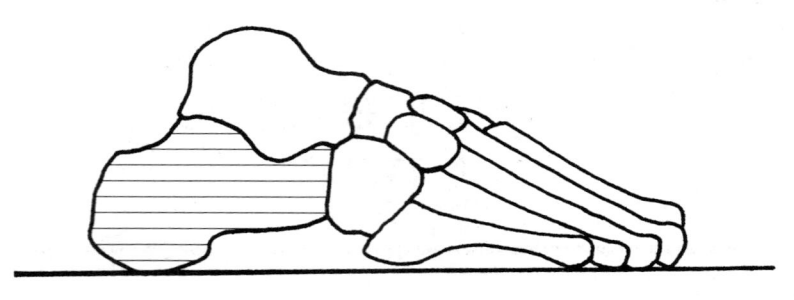

Figure 5.2.
With OKC STJ motion, only the calcaneus moves about the STJ axis.

5-6
Conversely, with OKC STJ supination, one would expect the calcaneus to _____, _____, and _____.

dorsiflexes

5-7
In OKC STJ motion, the calcaneus moves around the talus, which functions as an immobile extension of the leg. This contrasts with closed kinetic chain (CKC) STJ function in which both the talus and calcaneus move, albeit in different planes (Fig. 5.3).

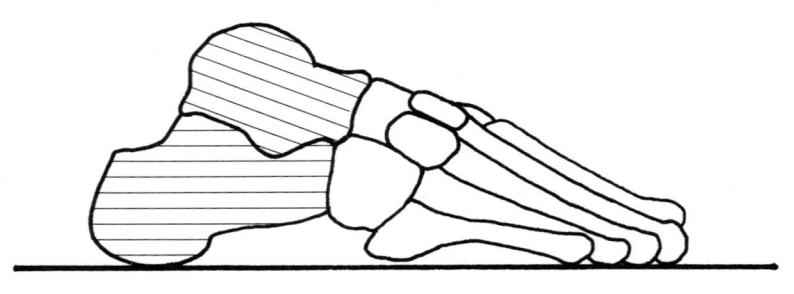

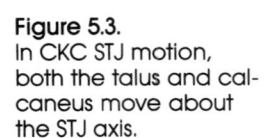

adduct, invert, plantarflex

Figure 5.3.
In CKC STJ motion, both the talus and calcaneus move about the STJ axis.

5-8
In OKC STJ motion, all elements of pronation or supination are exhibited exclusively by the _____.

calcaneus

5-9
Both the calcaneus and the talus move in (*OKC/CKC*) STJ motion.

CKC

5-10
The talus functions as an immobile extension of the leg in (*OKC/CKC*) STJ motion.

OKC

5-11
In OKC STJ pronation, the calcaneus moves around the talus in the directions of dorsiflexion, _____, and _____.

abduction, eversion

5-12
In CKC STJ motion, the calcaneus and talus both move. The calcaneus *only* moves in the *frontal plane*. Frontal plane motions are _____ and _____.

5: SUBTALAR JOINT FUNCTION IN OPEN AND CLOSED KINETIC CHAIN

inversion, eversion

5-13
In CKC STJ motion, the calcaneus only moves in the _____ plane.

frontal

5-14
This means that during CKC STJ motion, the talus must move in the _____ and _____ planes.

transverse, sagittal

5-15
The bones of the STJ move around the STJ's axis of motion. In OKC STJ pronation, this means that the calcaneus, which is *distal* to the axis, moves in all of the pronatory directions—i.e., abduction, eversion, and dorsiflexion.

If any motion takes places in a bone which is *proximal* to that axis, the motion will be in the *opposite* direction of the named major motion.

So, in CKC STJ pronation, the calcaneus will still evert, but the talus will exhibit opposite directional components of pronation in the sagittal and horizontal planes. That is to say the talus will plantarflex and adduct (Fig. 5.4).

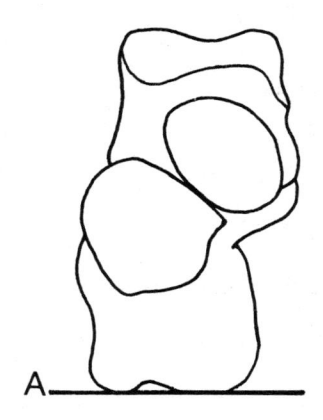

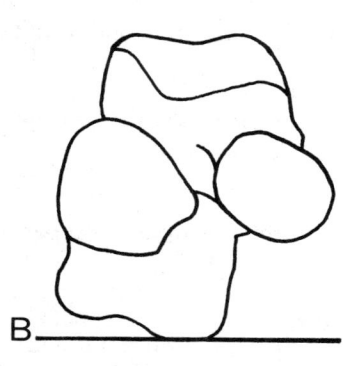

Figure 5.4.
A, The STJ in its neutral position. B, In CKC STJ pronation, the calcaneus everts while the talus adducts and plantarflexes.

5-16
Just remember that in CKC STJ motion, since the calcaneus is *distal* to the STJ axis, it will do what we expect it to do in the plane in which it moves—the _____ plane.

frontal

5-17
So, with CKC STJ supination, the calcaneus will exhibit (*inversion/eversion*).

inversion

5-18
And since the talus is proximal to the STJ axis of motion, with CKC STJ supination, it will _____ and _____.

dorsiflex, abduct

5-19
During the contact period, the STJ undergoes CKC _____.

pronation

5-20
This means that the calcaneus is _____ing while the talus is _____ing and _____ing.

evert, plantarflex, adduct	**5-21** Conversely, during the midstance and propulsive periods of the _____ phase of gait, one would normally observe the calcaneus to invert while the talus abducts and dorsiflexes. This occurs because the STJ is undergoing CKC _____.
stance, supination	**5-22** During the second half of the swing phase of gait, the STJ undergoes (*OKC/CKC*) (*pronation/supination*) (Fig. 5.5).

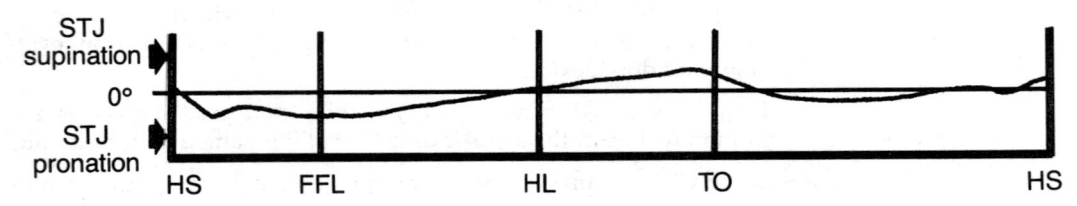

Figure 5.5. STJ motion during the gait cycle.

OKC supination	**5-23** This occurs in order for the foot to become more stable as it approaches heel strike. During this time, one would observe the talus to be _____.
immobile	**5-24** Simultaneously, the calcaneus would be _____ing, _____ing, and _____ing.
plantarflex, adduct, invert	**5-25** During the midstance period, however, the calcaneus would be _____ing only.
invert	**5-26** So, to review, during the first half of the swing phase of gait, the STJ exhibits (*OKC/CKC*) (*pronation/supination*).
OKC pronation	**5-27** During the last half of the swing phase, the STJ exhibits (*OKC/CKC*) (*pronation/supination*).
OKC supination	**5-28** During OKC STJ supination, which bone(s) move(s) and in which direction(s)?
calcaneus plantarflexes, inverts, and adducts	**5-29** During CKC STJ pronation, which bone(s) move(s) and in which direction(s)?

calcaneus everts, talus plantarflexes and adducts

5-30
An important point to consider is that tibial rotations are intimately related to CKC STJ motion. It has been observed that *with CKC STJ pronation, the tibia rotates internally* (Fig. 5.6).

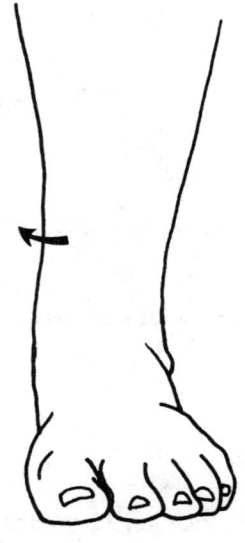

Figure 5.6.
Internal rotation of the tibia is observed with CKC STJ pronation.

5-31
The converse is true. That is, with CKC STJ supination, the tibia rotates _____ (Fig. 5.7).

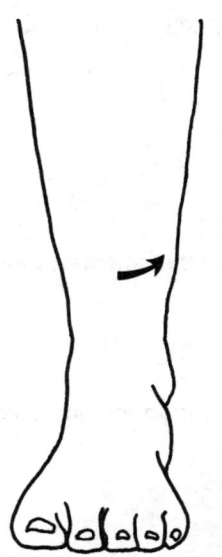

Figure 5.7.
With CKC STJ supination, the tibia rotates externally.

externally

5-32
If a patient were observed to have *excessive* internal tibial rotation during gait, then one might suspect a possible etiology to be excessive CKC STJ _____.

pronation

5-33
This completes the chapter on Subtalar Joint Function in Open and Closed Kinetic Chain. The next chapter is on Normal STJ Function in the Gait Cycle and will help to integrate the last two chapters.

Questions

FRAME 5-5

1. In *OKC STJ pronation*, the calcaneus exhibits:
    a. eversion
    b. abduction
    c. dorsiflexion
    d. a and b
    e. a, b, and c

FRAME 5-7

2. In *CKC* function, the talus functions as an immobile extension of the leg.
    a. true
    b. false

FRAME 5-12

3. With regard to *CKC* STJ function, the calcaneus moves in which plane(s)?
    a. sagittal
    b. frontal
    c. transverse
    d. a and b
    e. a and c

FRAME 5-15

4. In *CKC STJ pronation*, the calcaneus will evert and the talus will abduct and dorsiflex.
    a. true
    b. false

FRAME 5-21

5. During the *contact period*, the calcaneus normally:
    a. plantarflexes
    b. dorsiflexes
    c. supinates
    d. inverts
    e. everts

FRAME 5-23

6. During the second half of the swing phase, the STJ undergoes:
    a. OKC supination
    b. OKC pronation
    c. CKC pronation
    d. CKC supination
    e. none of the above

5: SUBTALAR JOINT FUNCTION IN OPEN AND CLOSED KINETIC CHAIN

7. With *CKC STJ pronation*, the tibia will:
   a. invert
   b. evert
   c. rotate externally
   d. rotate internally
   e. dorsiflex

8. The calcaneus everts while the talus plantarflexes and adducts during the entire:
   a. contact period
   b. midstance period
   c. propulsive period
   d. a and b
   e. b and c

9. In *CKC pronation*, the talus exhibits *opposite* directional components of supination in the sagittal and horizontal planes.
   a. true
   b. false

10. The talus functions as an immobile extension of the leg during the:
    a. contact period
    b. midstance period
    c. propulsive period
    d. stance phase
    e. swing phase

Answers

1. e
2. b
3. b
4. b
5. e
6. a
7. d
8. a
9. b
10. e

CHAPTER 6

Normal Subtalar Joint Function in the Gait Cycle

- subtalar joint (STJ) neutral position within the gait cycle
- STJ motion, position, and function during the contact period
- STJ motion, position, and function during the midstance period
- STJ motion, position, and function during the propulsive period
- STJ motion, position, and function during the swing phase
- relationship of tibial rotations to STJ motion

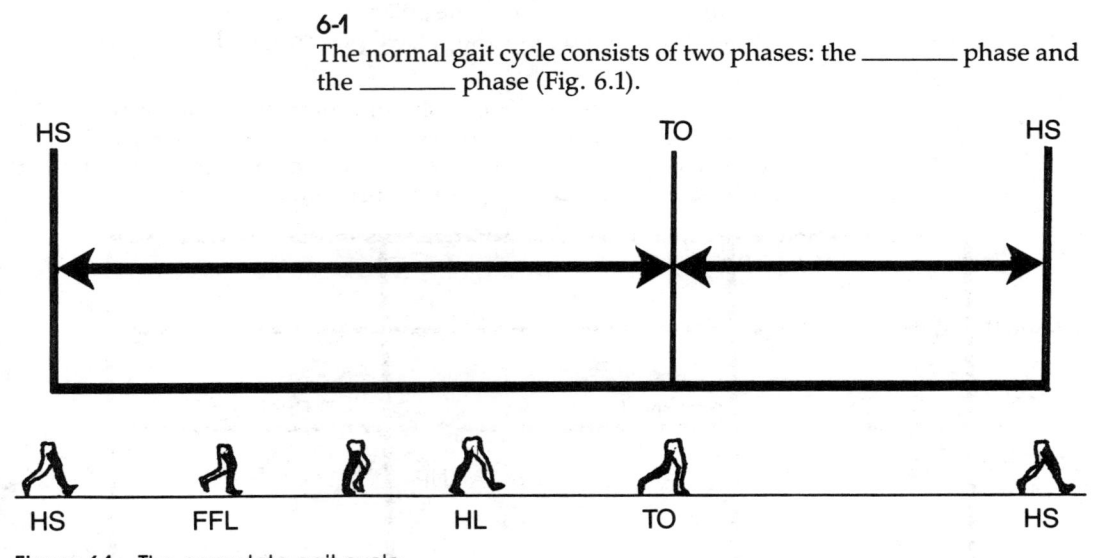

6-1
The normal gait cycle consists of two phases: the _____ phase and the _____ phase (Fig. 6.1).

Figure 6.1. The complete gait cycle.

stance, swing

6-2
Open Kinetic Chain (OKC) STJ function is observed during the _____ phase.

swing

6-3
During the first half of the swing phase (i.e., through midswing), the STJ exhibits OKC (*pronation/supination*).

FOOT FUNCTION: A PROGRAMMED TEXT

pronation

6-4
Soon after the swing phase begins and OKC STJ _____ starts, the STJ *position* becomes *pronated*.

pronation

6-5
Both the *motion of pronation* and the *pronated position* of the STJ occur so that the foot may clear the ground as the lower extremity swings forward.

Additionally, the *energy* expended to accomplish ground clearance is minimized by STJ pronation. Without STJ pronation allowing the STJ to achieve a pronated position, it would be necessary to use the hip and thigh musculature even more to accomplish the same ground clearance.

6-6
During the last half of the swing phase (i.e., after STJ OKC pronation), the STJ exhibits (*OKC/CKC*) (*pronation/supination*).

OKC supination

6-7
This supination occurs so that the foot will become more stable in preparation for heel strike.

6-8
With the STJ, we know that the point in an ideal foot which separates a pronated position from a supinated position is called the STJ *neutral position*.

At heel strike, the STJ is in a slightly supinated position (Fig. 6.2). Since the STJ is in a pronated position at midswing and is in a slightly supinated position just after heel strike, we know that the STJ must have reached its _____ position just before heel strike.

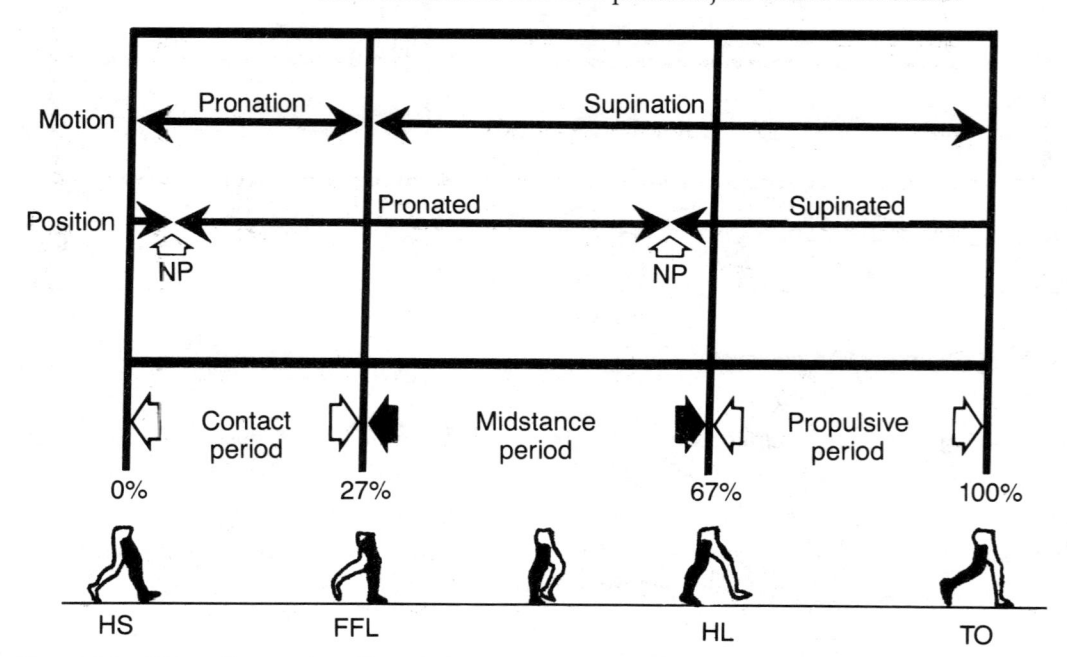

Figure 6.2. STJ motion and position during the gait cycle. NP refers to the STJ neutral position; HS = heel strike; FFL = forefoot loading; HL = heel lift; TO = toe off.

neutral	**6-9** Immediately after heel strike, the STJ exhibits (*OKC/CKC*) (*pronation/supination*).
CKC pronation	**6-10** This pronation brings the STJ first into its neutral position and then past it into a pronated position. Two major functions of this contact period CKC STJ pronation are to allow the foot to act as a *mobile adaptor* for terrain variances and to *absorb shock* as the body weight is transmitted through the lower extremity. At heel strike, the STJ is in a slightly _____ position.
supinated	**6-11** Recall that during the CKC STJ pronation of the contact period, the calcaneus is _____ing and the talus is _____ing and _____ing.
evert, adduct, plantar-flex	**6-12** The two major functions of the CKC STJ pronation during the contact period are to allow the foot to act as a _____ _____ and to absorb _____.
mobile adaptor, shock	**6-13** In patients who have had a triple arthrodesis of the STJ, the shock-absorbing function of the STJ is lost. Because of this, excessive shock is transmitted to the joints of the lower extremity and secondary degeneration of the ankle, knee, and/or hip joints may be seen several years after the surgery.

6-14
If biomechanical pathology exists which prevents the normal contact period CKC STJ pronation from occurring, one might expect to see a(an) (*increase/decrease*) in normal shock absorption. This may lead to degenerative changes in the joints of the lower extremity (Fig. 6.3). Additionally, a significantly decreased ability to accommodate variances in terrain would be observed.

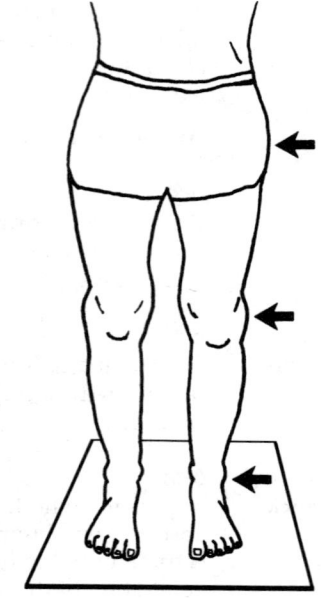

Figure 6.3.
Diminished or absent contact period STJ pronation can lead to degenerative changes in the ankle, knee, and hip. The ability to accommodate for terrain variances would also be diminished.

decrease

6-15
During the first half of the swing phase, the STJ exhibits _____ _____.

OKC pronation

6-16
After the midswing point and through heel strike, the STJ exhibits _____ _____.

OKC supination

6-17
During the contact period, the STJ undergoes _____ _____.

CKC pronation

6-18
The two major functions of contact period CKC STJ pronation are: _____ _____ and adapting to terrain variances.

shock absorption

6-19
During the contact period, the calcaneus _____ while the talus _____ and _____.

everts, adducts, plantarflexes

6-20
At midstance, which begins with _____ _____ of the _____ foot, the STJ begins undergoing CKC _____.

6: NORMAL SUBTALAR JOINT FUNCTION IN THE GAIT CYCLE

toe off, opposite, supination

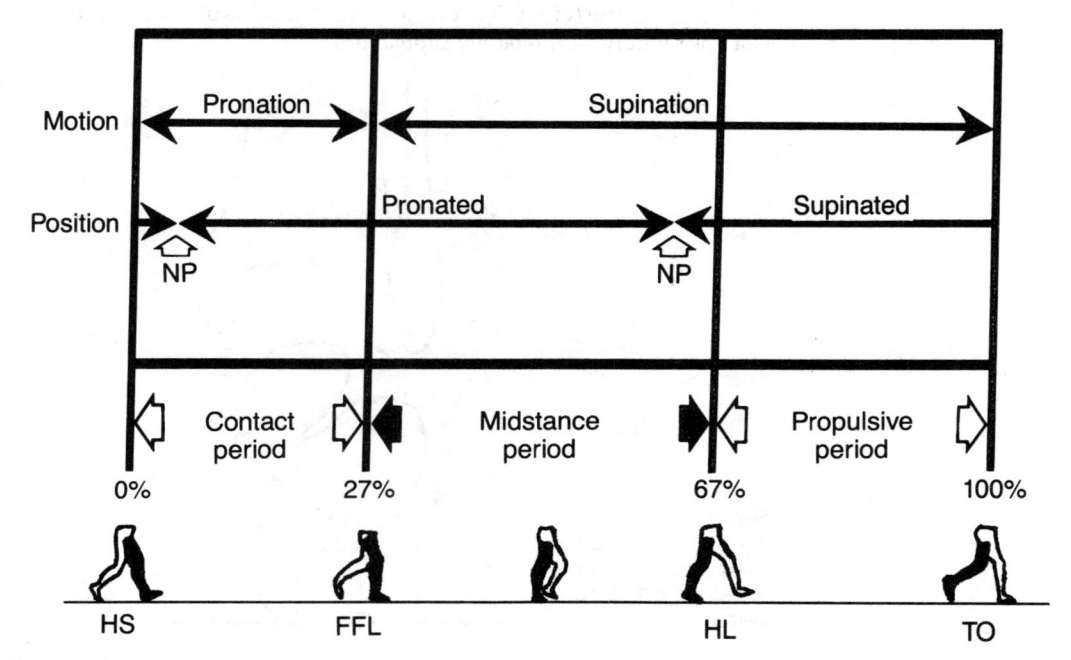

6-21
Even though the STJ is supinating throughout midstance, it is in a pronated *position* until just before heel lift when it reaches its neutral position (Fig. 6.4). The other time during the stance phase when the STJ reached its neutral position was just after _____ _____.

Figure 6.4.
STJ motion and position during the gait cycle.

heel strike

6-22
Heel strike and *heel* lift have the STJ neutral position in common.

6-23
So, the STJ reaches its neutral position at two points during the stance phase of gait. The first time is just after heel strike and the last time is just before _____ _____ during the _____ period.

heel lift, midstance

6-24
During the midstance and propulsive periods, the progressive CKC STJ supination makes the foot into a more and more rigid lever in preparation for propelling the body forward at the end of the _____ period.

propulsive

6-25
During the midstance and propulsive periods, the calcaneus is _____ing while the talus is _____ing and _____ing.

invert, abduct, dorsiflex

6-26
The talus abducts and dorsiflexes during CKC STJ supination because it is _____ to the STJ joint axis.

proximal

6-27
In OKC STJ motion, the talus functions as an extension of the leg and does not move relative to STJ motion.

In CKC STJ motion, the talus moves with the tibia in the *transverse* plane. When the tibia rotates internally, the talus adducts in the transverse plane (Fig. 6.5). Adduction of the talus in CKC STJ motion is a component of (*pronation/supination*).

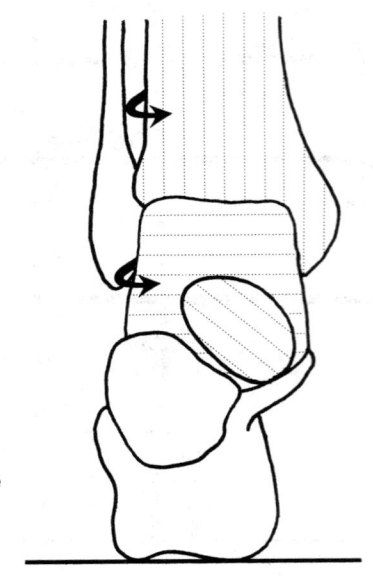

Figure 6.5.
In CKC STJ motion, the talus and tibia move together in the transverse plane.

pronation

6-28
If the tibia rotates _____ with CKC STJ pronation, it would be reasonable and, in fact, true to assume that *with CKC STJ supination, the tibia rotates externally.*

internally

6-29
So, since the talus moves with the tibia in CKC STJ motion, one would expect excessive CKC pronation to produce excessive (*internal/external*) tibial rotation. (Note that tibial rotation is a transverse plane motion.)

internal

6-30
Likewise, excessive external tibial rotation would be observed with excessive CKC STJ _____.

supination

6-31
In fact, one sees many more patients with excessive CKC STJ pronation causing excessive _____ tibial rotation.

internal

6-32
This excessive internal tibial rotation sometimes causes abnormally large forces to be exerted on the cartilaginous surfaces of the knee joint. It is not uncommon to see patients (especially runners) complaining of this type of knee problem secondary to this etiology—i.e., excessive CKC STJ _____.

6: NORMAL SUBTALAR JOINT FUNCTION IN THE GAIT CYCLE

pronation

6-33
It is easy to see that the STJ affects structures proximal to itself. The implications of abnormal STJ function not only include the joints and muscles of the foot but those of the knee, hip, and spine as well.

6-34
To review, during the first half of the swing phase, the STJ exhibits (*OKC/CKC*) (*pronation/supination*).

OKC pronation

6-35
From midswing to the end of the swing phase, the STJ exhibits (*OKC/CKC*) (*pronation/supination*).

OKC supination

6-36
The OKC STJ supination during the last half of the swing phase makes the foot (*more/less*) rigid as it prepares it for heel strike.

more

6-37
The OKC STJ pronation during the first half of the swing phase helps the foot to _____ the ground.

clear

6-38
At heel strike, the STJ is slightly (*pronated/supinated*).

supinated

6-39
Directly after heel strike, the STJ begins _____ which it continues throughout the contact period.

pronating

6-40
The two major functions of the contact period CKC STJ pronation are to _____ _____ and to allow the foot to act as a _____ _____ for terrain variances.

absorb shock, mobile adaptor

6-41
The first time during the stance phase that the STJ reaches it neutral position is just after _____ _____.

heel strike

6-42
After the beginning of the midstance period (which correlates with _____ _____ of the _____ foot), the STJ begins CKC _____.

toe off, opposite, supination

6-43
Does CKC supination continue throughout most of the propulsive period?

yes

6-44
The STJ reaches its neutral position for the second time during the stance phase just (*after/before*) heel lift.

before

6-45
The function of the progressive CKC STJ supination during the _____ and _____ periods is to make the foot into a more (*flexible/rigid*) lever.

midstance, propulsive, rigid	**6-46** During most of the propulsive period, the calcaneus is _____ing while the talus is _____ing and _____ing.
invert, abduct, dorsiflex	**6-47** During the midstance and propulsive periods, the tibia is _____ rotating as the STJ is _____ing.
externally, supinat(ing)	**6-48** In CKC, the talus and the tibia move together in the _____ plane.
transverse	**6-49** This completes Chapter 6. The next chapter will deal with the OKC measurement of and neutral position calculation for the STJ.

Questions

FRAME 6-4 AND 6-5

1. Soon after the swing phase begins the STJ position becomes pronated.
    a. true
    b. false

FRAME 6-8

2. At heel strike, the STJ is in what position?
    a. very pronated
    b. slightly pronated
    c. very supinated
    d. slightly supinated
    e. neutral

FRAME 6-10

3. Allowing the foot to act as a mobile adaptor and absorb shock are two specific major functions of the:
    a. contact period
    b. midstance period
    c. propulsive period
    d. swing phase
    e. talar cartilage

FRAME 6-21

4. The STJ reaches its neutral position toward the end of the midstance period after supinating throughout the midstance period.
    a. true
    b. false

5. The STJ reaches its neutral position during the stance phase just:
   a. after heel strike
   b. before heel strike
   c. before heel lift
   d. a and b
   e. a and c

FRAME 6-21 AND 6-23

6. In CKC STJ motion, the talus moves with the tibia in which plane?
   a. sagittal
   b. transverse
   c. frontal
   d. a, b, and c
   e. the talus does not move with the tibia in CKC function.

FRAME 6-27

7. Excessive CKC STJ pronation can cause:
   a. excessive internal tibial rotation
   b. excessive external tibial rotation
   c. knee symptoms
   d. a and c
   e. b and c

FRAMES 6-29–6-32

8. The talus functions as an extension of the leg and does not move relative to STJ motion in:
   a. OKC supination
   b. CKC supination
   c. OKC pronation
   d. a and b
   e. a and c

FRAME 6-27

9. The talus abducts and dorsiflexes in CKC STJ pronation.
   a. true
   b. false

FRAME 6-26

10. During the midstance and propulsive periods, progressive CKC STJ supination makes the foot into a progressively more rigid lever.
    a. true
    b. false

FRAME 6-24

Answers

1. a	4. a	7. d	10. a
2. d	5. e	8. e	
3. a	6. b	9. b	

CHAPTER 7

Subtalar Joint—Open Kinetic Chain Measurement and Neutral Position Calculation

- clinical index of STJ motion—definition and measurement
- normal motion from the STJ neutral position
- average total STJ range of motion
- minimum necessary STJ range of motion for normal ambulation
- measurements for determining STJ neutral position
- calculation of STJ neutral position

7-1
Motion which occurs around the STJ axis is (*mono/bi/tri*)plane motion.

tri

7-2
Clinically, there is no good way to measure the STJ motion in all three planes.

Instead, we use the *frontal plane motion of the calcaneus*, a bone (*proximal/distal*) to the STJ axis, as an *index of STJ motion* (Fig. 7.1).

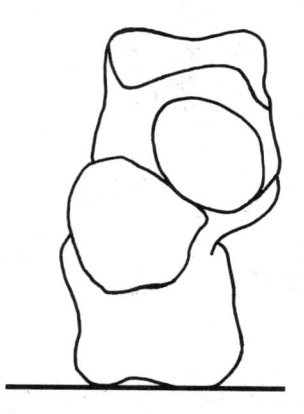

Figure 7.1.
An anterior view of the STJ. The frontal plane motion of the calcaneus is used as an index of STJ motion.

distal	**7-3** Since the calcaneus is distal to the axis of the STJ, with *CKC* pronation it will _____.
evert	**7-4** Likewise, the frontal plane motion of the calcaneus with *OKC* pronation is _____.
eversion	**7-5** So, in both weightbearing and non-weightbearing situations, the calcaneus will _____ with pronation and _____ with supination.
evert, invert	**7-6** As an index of STJ motion, we measure the motion of the calcaneus in the _____ plane. *It is common to refer to the degrees of calcaneal inversion and eversion when talking about the total STJ ROM. Even though we are actually talking about calcaneal motion in the frontal plane, in this one special instance, we may use inversion interchangeably with supination and eversion interchangeably with pronation.*
frontal	**7-7** The STJ position between a supinated and pronated position of a normal foot (Fig. 7.2) is called the _____ position.

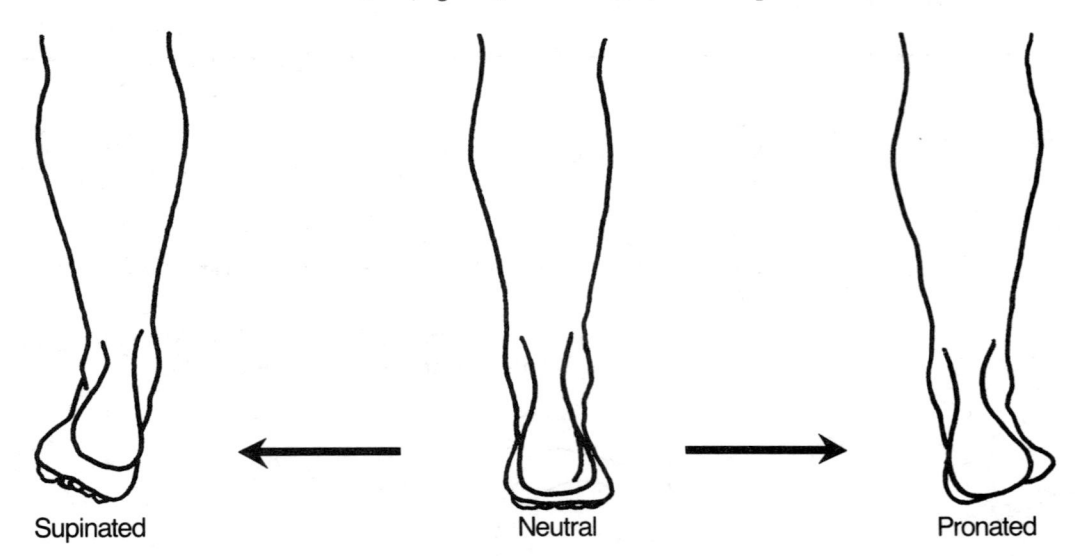

Figure 7.2. The STJ neutral position is found between the supinated and pronated STJ positions.

neutral	**7-8** At the neutral position of the STJ, the foot is neither supinated nor _____.

7: SUBTALAR JOINT—OPEN KINETIC CHAIN MEASUREMENT AND NEUTRAL POSITION CALCULATION

7-9

pronated

From the STJ neutral position, the normal foot can supinate twice as much as it can pronate (Fig. 7.3). Therefore, when we measure the frontal plane motion of the calcaneus to assess the STJ motion, we would expect there to be two times as much _____ as there is _____.

Supinated   Neutral   Pronated

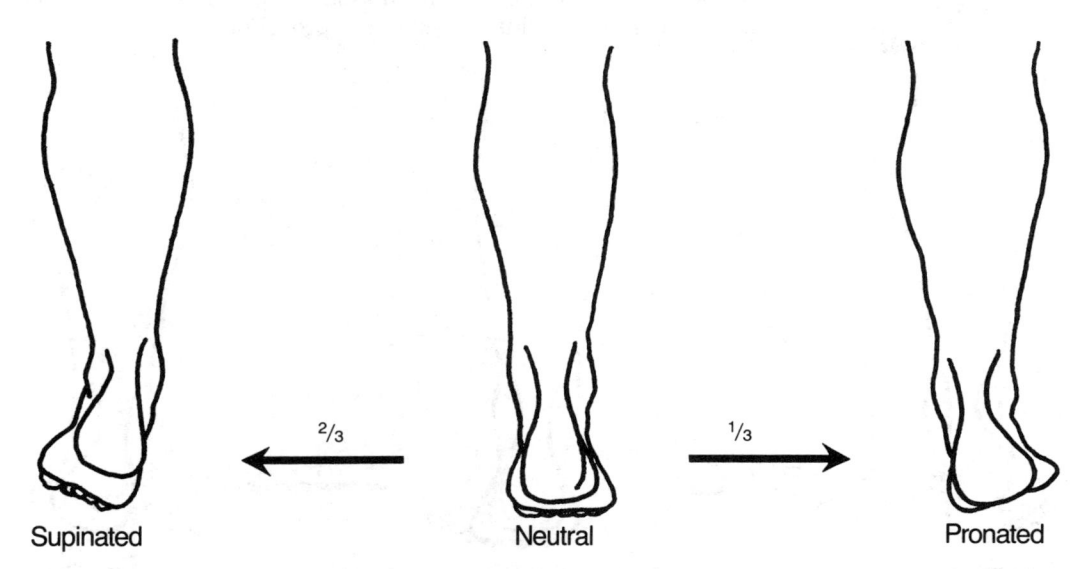

Figure 7.3. Two-thirds of the STJ motion is in a supinatory direction, while the remaining one-third is in a pronatory direction. The STJ can, therefore, supinate twice as many degrees as it can pronate.

7-10

inversion/supination, eversion/pronation

The *average* total range of motion (ROM) for the STJ is about *30°* of calcaneal frontal plane motion (as observed clinically).

7-11

If a patient had 30° of motion (the _____ total ROM for the STJ), we would expect to see 10° of pronation from the neutral position and 20° of supination from the neutral position (Fig. 7.4).

This would be expected in the normal foot because the STJ has _____ as much supination as it does pronation.

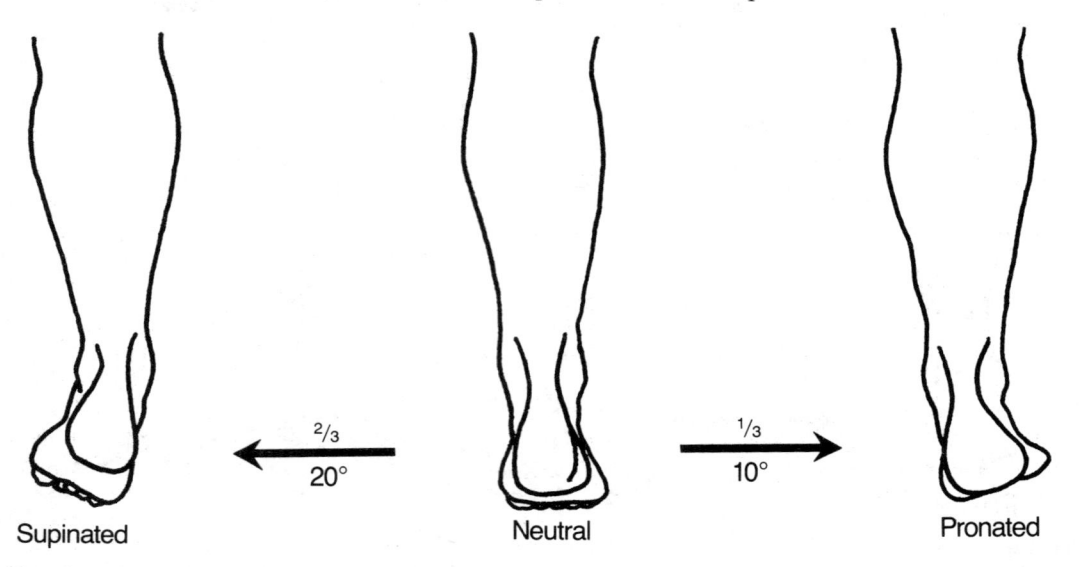

Figure 7.4.

Supinated — 2/3 — 20° ← Neutral → 1/3 — 10° — Pronated

average, twice

7-12

Another way of saying this is that the total STJ motion is composed of one-third pronation and two-thirds supination.

7-13

The *average* measured ROM for the STJ is about _____° of calcaneal _____ plane motion.

30, frontal

7-14

While 30° of calcaneal frontal plane motion is the average normal index of total STJ motion, the minimum total STJ ROM necessary for normal ambulation is 8° to 12°.

For our purposes, we will simplify this figure and say that *the minimum total STJ ROM necessary for normal ambulation is 10°*.

7-15

The *average* total STJ ROM clinically observed is about _____°.

The *minimum* total STJ ROM necessary for normal ambulation is _____°.

These degrees are measured in the _____ plane with calcaneal motion.

7: SUBTALAR JOINT—OPEN KINETIC CHAIN MEASUREMENT AND NEUTRAL POSITION CALCULATION

30, 10, frontal

7-16
In order to appreciate what normal STJ motion and function should be for a given patient, the STJ neutral position must be calculated from non-weightbearing (i.e., OKC) measurements taken during the biomechanical examination of the lower extremity.

The OKC measurements used for this purpose are *inversion and eversion of the calcaneus relative to the distal one-third of the leg*. For this measurement, marks are used which bisect the posterior aspect of the calcaneus and the posterior aspect of the distal one-third of the leg (Fig. 7.5).

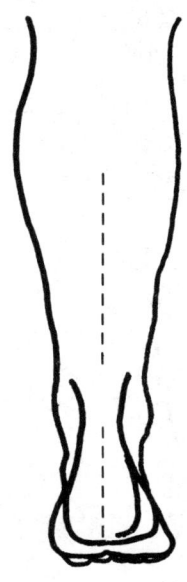

Figure 7.5.
Bisections of the posterior aspects of the leg and calcaneus are used for the clinical measurements of the STJ.

7-17
To determine the STJ's neutral position, we used (*CKC/OKC*) measurements of calcaneal _____ plane motion relative to the (*proximal/distal*) one-third of the leg.

OKC, frontal, distal

7-18
To facilitate this measurement, marks are used which _____ the posterior distal one-third of the leg and the _____.

bisect, calcaneus

7-19
Recall that the normal STJ has a total ROM composed of (*one-third/two-thirds*) pronation and (*one-third/two-thirds*) supination.

one-third, two-thirds

7-20

In a non-weightbearing patient, the bisection of the posterior distal one-third of the leg is the point from which calcaneal inversion and eversion are measured.

Assume that a calcaneus can evert 8° from the leg bisection and invert 22° from the leg bisection (Fig. 7.6). The total STJ ROM is 30° (inversion + eversion), but there would be only 8° of eversion and 22° of inversion from the leg bisection.

To obtain the neutral position of this STJ, we need to find the point from which there is twice as much supination as there is pronation. In this case, the neutral position would be 2° inverted (relative to the leg bisection). From this point, there is 10° of pronation available and 20° of supination available. Thus, it has fulfilled the rule that the STJ has one-third pronatory motion and two-thirds supinatory motion available from its neutral position.

This is a concept that you may want to reread once or twice before going on.

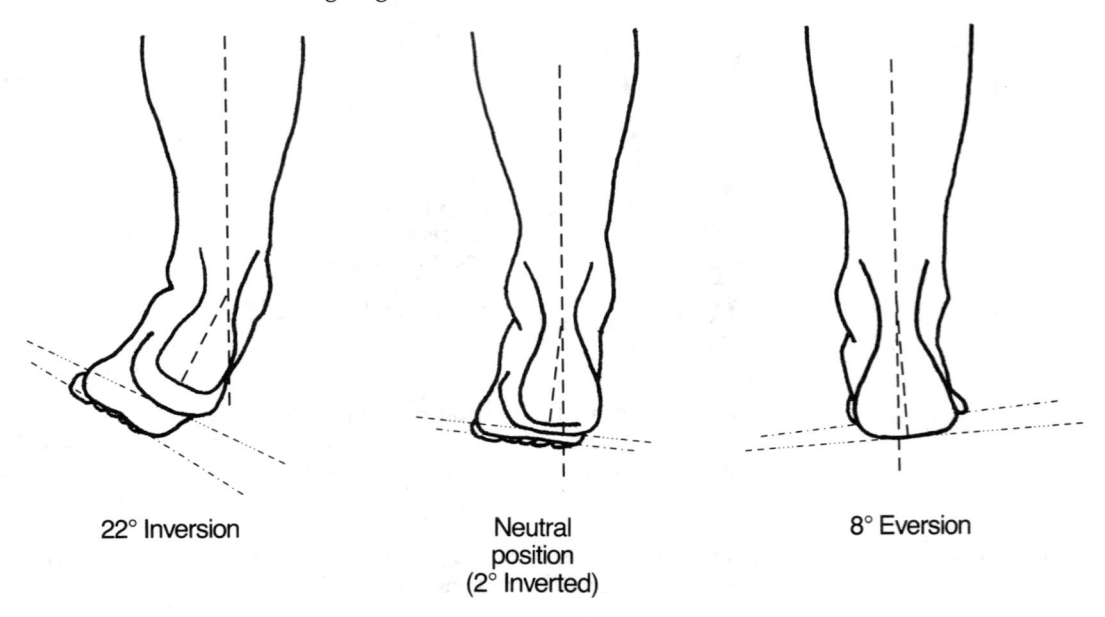

22° Inversion   Neutral position (2° Inverted)   8° Eversion

Figure 7.6.

7-21

A cookbook method of calculating the neutral position of the STJ is to subtract the *amount of calcaneal eversion available from the STJ neutral position* from the *calcaneal eversion available from the leg bisection*.

In the above example we had:

8° of calcaneal eversion from the leg bisection available
10° of calcaneal eversion from the STJ neutral position available (total STJ ROM was 30° and eversion motion = one-third of the total)

Subtracting (8° − 10°), we get a remainder of −2°.

The minus sign means that the position is inverted. (Conversely, a positive number means that the position is everted.)

Thus, the STJ neutral position in this example would be 2° *inverted*.

7: SUBTALAR JOINT—OPEN KINETIC CHAIN MEASUREMENT AND NEUTRAL POSITION CALCULATION

7-22
The STJ neutral position will always be that point from which there is *(twice/half)* as much pronatory motion as there is supinatory motion.

half

7-23
Here is a problem for you to try:

On OKC examination, you find that a patient has:

7° of calcaneal eversion from the leg bisection
20° of calcaneal inversion from the leg bisection
(Total STJ ROM = _____°)

Therefore, the amount of pronation available from the neutral position must be _____° and the amount of supination available from the neutral position is _____°.

By subtracting as described above, you get a remainder of _____° which translates into a neutral position of _____° *(inverted/everted)* from the leg bisection.

27, 9, 18, −2, 2°, inverted

7-24
The key in this calculation is to be aware of how much pronatory (or supinatory) motion is available from the STJ neutral position. Once you know this, you can pretty well see if the neutral position should be inverted or everted relative to the leg bisection.

7-25
Here is one last problem before we review this chapter:

On examination, you find the following (Fig. 7.7):

8° of calcaneal eversion from the leg bisection
16° of calcaneal inversion from the leg bisection
Total STJ ROM = _____°

Therefore, the amount of pronation available from the STJ's neutral position is _____° and the amount of supination available from the neutral position is _____°.

By subtracting as described, you get a remainder of _____.

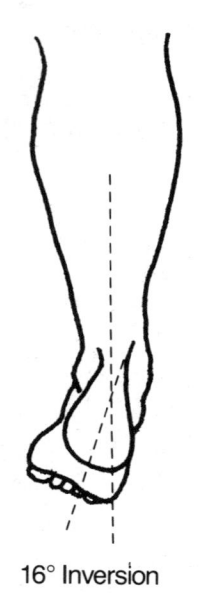

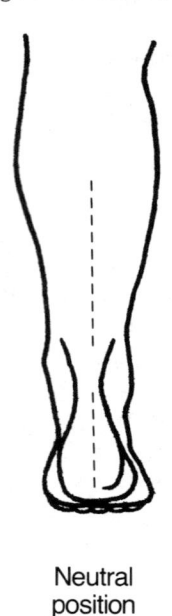

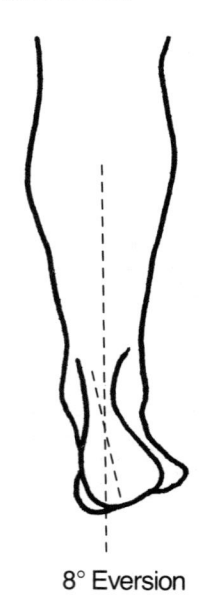

16° Inversion   Neutral position   8° Eversion

Figure 7.7.

24, 8, 16, 0

7-26
The remainder of 0 means that the STJ neutral position is parallel with the leg bisection.

In this case, we would state that the STJ neutral position equals 0 degrees.

7-27
As an index of STJ triplane motion, we use the _____ plane motion of the _____.

frontal, calcaneus

7-28
Only when discussing STJ motion, therefore, can we use calcaneal inversion interchangeably with STJ _____ and calcaneal eversion interchangeably with STJ _____.

supination, pronation

7-29
The *average* total STJ ROM observed clinically is _____° of calcaneal frontal plane motion.

30	**7-30** The *minimum* total STJ ROM necessary for normal ambulation is _____°.
10	**7-31** Of the total STJ ROM, pronation composes (*one-third/two-thirds*) and supination composes (*one-third/two-thirds*).
one-third, two-thirds	**7-32** To determine the STJ neutral position, calcaneal motion in the frontal plane is measured relative to the _____ _____-_____ of the leg.
distal one-third	**7-33** This motion is measured clinically by measuring marks which _____ the posterior aspects of the distal one-third of the leg and the _____.
bisect, calcaneus	**7-34** The STJ has _____ as much supinatory motion as it does pronatory motion as measured from its _____ position.
twice, neutral	**7-35** This completes the chapter. In the next two chapters, we will examine factors which affect rearfoot position and the weightbearing assessment of the STJ. Following those is a chapter which lets you solve (through calculation and interpretation) case histories involving STJ pathology.

Questions

FRAME 7-2

1. The *index* of STJ motion that is used clinically is the:
    a. sagittal plane motion of the calcaneus
    b. frontal plane motion of the calcaneus
    c. transverse plane motion of the calcaneus
    d. transverse plane motion of the talus
    e. frontal plane motion of the talus

FRAME 7-5

2. In *OKC* supination, the calcaneus _____, and in *CKC* supination, it _____.
    a. adducts, adducts
    b. adducts, abducts
    c. abducts, abducts
    d. inverts, everts
    e. inverts, inverts

FRAMES 7-7 AND 7-8

3. The foot is either pronated or supinated when the STJ is in its neutral position.
   a. true
   b. false

FRAME 7-9

4. From its neutral position, the STJ can supinate _____ as much as it can pronate.
   a. equally
   b. one-half
   c. one-third
   d. two-thirds
   e. twice

FRAME 7-10

5. The *average* total STJ ROM as measured in degrees of calcaneal frontal plane motion is:
   a. 10°
   b. 15°
   c. 20°
   d. 25°
   e. 30°

FRAME 7-13

6. The *minimum* total STJ ROM necessary for normal ambulation is:
   a. 10°
   b. 15°
   c. 20°
   d. 25°
   e. 30°

FRAME 7-16

7. To determine the STJ neutral position, *CKC* measurements are used.
   a. true
   b. false

FRAME 7-22

8. While performing an OKC examination, you find that a patient has the following:
   7° of calcaneal eversion from the leg bisection
   20° of calcaneal inversion from the leg bisection
   What do you calculate the STJ neutral position to be?
   a. 9° inverted
   b. 9° everted
   c. 2° everted
   d. 2° inverted
   e. 0°

FRAMES 7-19 AND 7-20

9. While performing an OKC examination, you find that a patient has the following:
   8° calcaneal eversion from the leg bisection
   22° calcaneal inversion from the leg bisection
   What do you calculate the neutral position of the STJ to be?
   a. 10° inverted
   b. 10° everted
   c. 2° inverted
   d. 2° everted
   e. 0°

FRAME 7-12

10. The total STJ ROM is composed of one-third pronation and two-thirds supination.
   a. true
   b. false

Answers

1. b
2. e
3. b
4. e
5. e
6. a
7. b
8. d
9. c
10. a

CHAPTER 8

Factors Affecting Rearfoot Position

- STJ axis and its relationship to adjacent muscles
- pronators and supinators of the STJ
- effect of muscular dysfunction on rearfoot position
- Charcot-Marie-Tooth disease
- peroneal spastic flatfoot
- subtalar varus and valgus
- rearfoot varus and valgus
- tibial varum and valgum
- tarsal coalition

8-1
The "normal foot" (see Appendix II) is rarely seen clinically. This is particularly true with regard to rearfoot position (as measured by the bisection of the posterior calcaneus relative to the posterior bisection of the distal one-third of the _____).

leg

8-2
Any muscular dysfunction which alters the balance between pronators and supinators of the STJ has the capacity to affect rearfoot position. This is true whether the dysfunction be *paretic* or *tonically spastic* in nature.

(The number of muscle disorders that can be responsible for abnormal rearfoot position are numerous. To appreciate the concepts, we will examine one disease from each category.)

8-3
Before we discuss the effect that muscle imbalance may have on the STJ, it is a good idea to review the spatial orientation of the STJ axis.

Recall that the STJ axis is oriented _____° from the *sagittal* plane and forty-*t*wo degrees from the _____ plane.

8-4

16, transverse | Additionally, the STJ axis runs from (HINT: dentist's degree) _____, _____, and _____ to _____, _____, and _____ (Fig. 8.1).

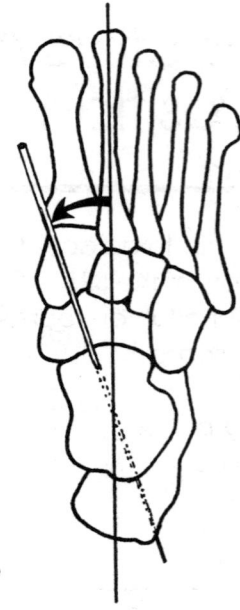

Figure 8.1.
A dorsal view of the STJ axis.

8-5

distal, medial, dorsal, proximal, lateral, plantar | Any muscle that runs *medial* to this axis will be a *supinator* of the STJ.

Examples of muscles which are STJ supinators are all of the muscles of the posterior leg which cross the STJ—the *gastrocnemius* and *soleus*, the *posterior tibial*, and the *long digital flexors*.

On the anterior aspect of the leg, the *anterior tibial* muscle supinates the STJ.

8-6

STJ supinators are muscles which run _____ to the STJ axis.

The STJ axis is angulated 16° from the _____ plane and _____° from the _____ plane.

8-7

medial, sagittal, 42, transverse | Specific muscles which supinate the STJ—located in the posterior leg—are the long digital _____, the _____ _____, and the gastrocnemius and _____.

8-8

flexors, posterior tibial, soleus | On the anterior leg, the muscle which supinates the STJ is the _____ _____.

8-9

anterior tibial | If one or more of these muscles contract insufficiently to balance the pronators, then the foot will be pulled into a pronated position.

8: FACTORS AFFECTING REARFOOT POSITION

8-10

Conversely, if the pronators of the STJ become weakened, the foot will assume a supinated attitude (e.g., pes cavus).

Pronators of the STJ cross *laterally* to that joint.

The pronators of the STJ are the *peroneals* (brevis and longus) as well as the *extensor digitorum longus* (with the *peroneus tertius*).

8-11

In Charcot-Marie-Tooth disease, there is progressive atrophy (and paresis) of the peroneal musculature (Fig. 8.2). Since the peroneals are _____ of the STJ, the foot would progressively assume a more _____ attitude.

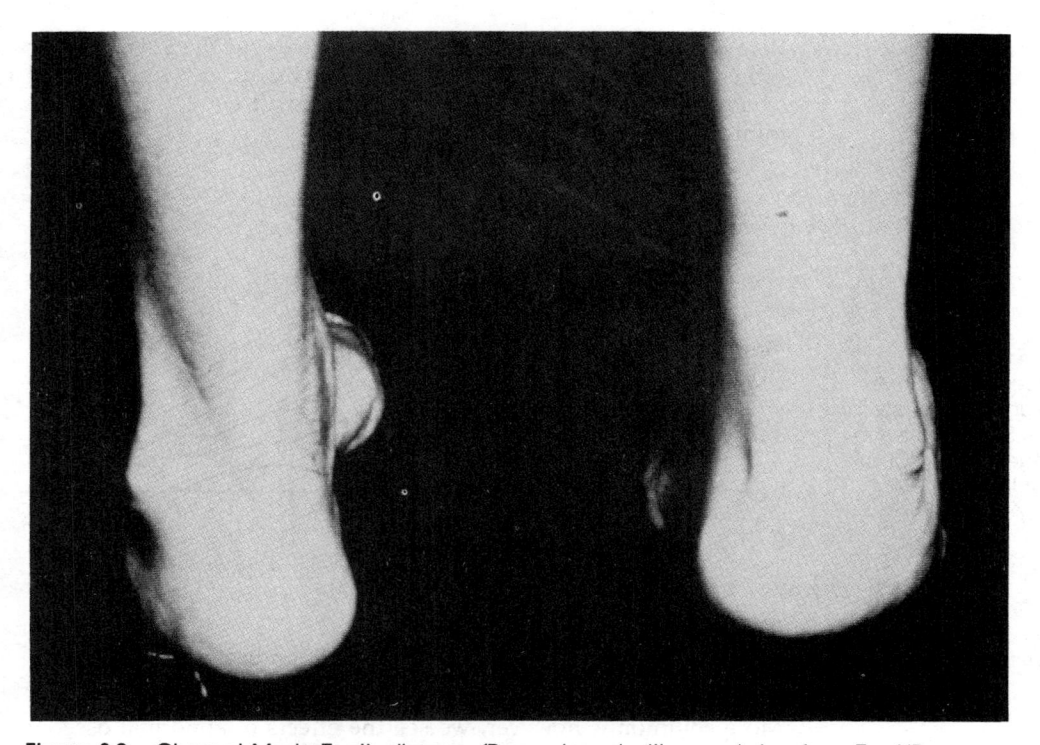

Figure 8.2. Charcot-Marie-Tooth disease. (Reproduced with permission from Tax HR: *Podopediatrics,* ed. 2. Baltimore, Williams & Wilkins, 1985, p 145.)

pronators, supinated

8-12

Besides the peroneus longus and brevis, other pronators of the STJ are the _____ _____ _____ and the peroneus _____.

extensor digitorum longus, tertius

8-13

Supinators of the STJ include the _____ and soleus, the _____ _____, and the long _____ _____.

gastrocnemius, posterior tibial, digital flexors

8-14
One of the most common muscles to be involved in spastically altering STJ position is the *peroneus brevis* (Fig. 8.3), the *strongest pronator of the STJ*.

This is the muscle which, in chronic spasm, causes peroneal spastic flatfoot. (There may be an associated peroneus longus spasm as well.)

The etiology of the spasm is most frequently an inflammatory condition in or around the STJ and/or MTJ.

(TREATMENT NOTE: A peroneal nerve block will relieve the spasm and secondary pronated position of the foot in peroneal spastic flatfoot.)

Recall that if STJ pronation is not available (because the STJ is already pronated) at and after heel strike, the ability to absorb _____ and to adapt the foot for variances in terrain will be significantly diminished.

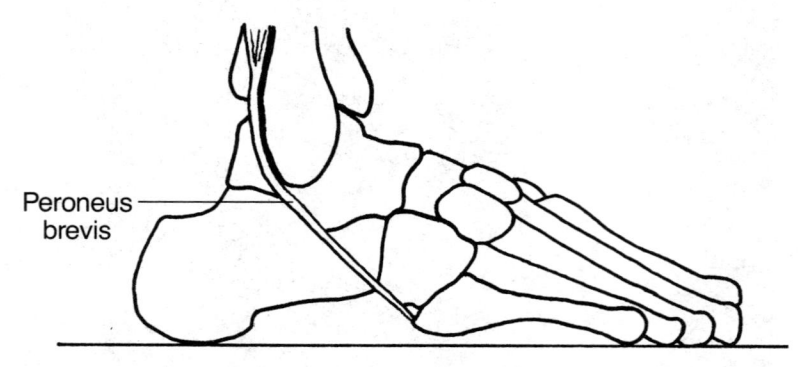

Figure 8.3.
The peroneus brevis runs and inserts lateral to the STJ axis. It is the strongest pronator of the STJ.

shock

peroneus brevis

8-15
The strongest pronator of the STJ is the _____ _____.

8-16
So, we have seen how spasm and paresis of muscles which run medial and lateral to the STJ can abnormally alter the rearfoot position.

More commonly, however, we see the effects of abnormal osseous structure on the STJ position. In this chapter, we will limit the remainder of the discussion to the femur, tibia, and the articular components of the STJ—the talus and the _____.

The effects of the forefoot and MTJ on STJ position will be discussed in later chapters.

calcaneus

8-17

A normal STJ neutral position is one in which the *posterior calcaneal bisection is parallel to the posterior bisection of the distal one-third of the leg* (Fig. 8.4).

Additionally, we know that from the STJ neutral position, there is a given amount of supination, the degrees of which are equal to (*one-half/twice*) the amount of pronation available from that position.

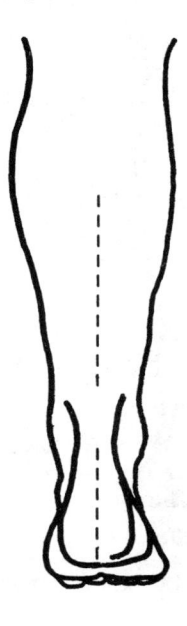

Figure 8.4.
When the normal STJ is in its neutral position, the calcaneal bisector is parallel to the posterior bisection of the distal one-third of the leg.

twice

8-18

We can then identify a "normal" STJ neutral position by the fact that there is (*one-half/twice*) the amount of pronation available from that point as there is supination (Fig. 8.5).

We can also identify a normal STJ neutral position by the observation that the calcaneal bisector is (*inverted/parallel/everted*) to the leg bisector.

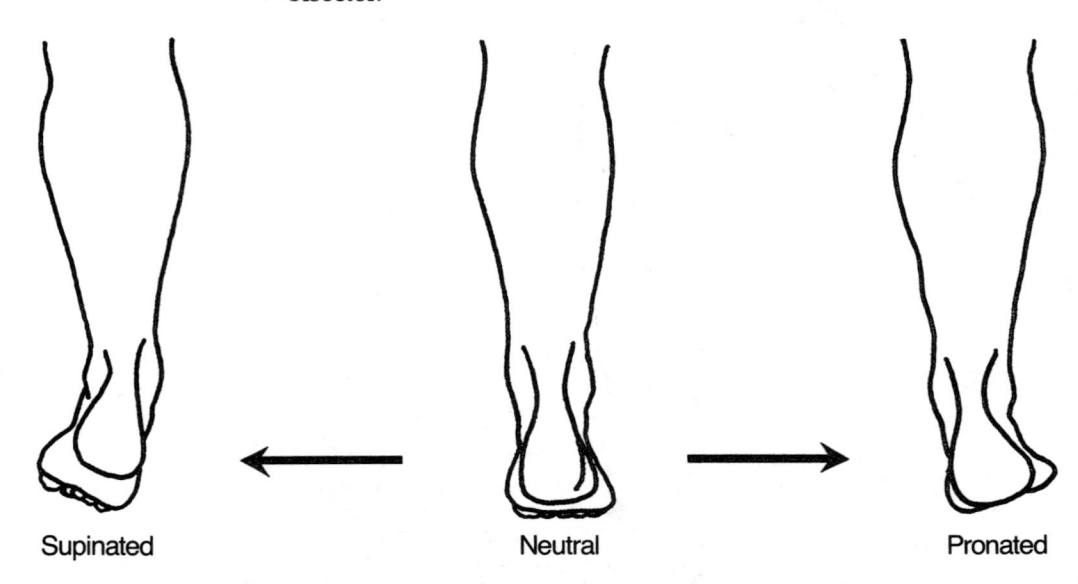

Supinated   Neutral   Pronated

Figure 8.5. The STJ neutral position can be identified by the relative amounts of motion away from it in pronatory and supinatory directions as well as the relationship of calcaneal and leg bisectors.

one-half, parallel

8-19

When the neutral position of the STJ is altered from the normal parallel relationship *between the calcaneus and the leg,* we define this as *subtalar varus* or *subtalur valgus.*

Subtalar valugs is defined as *a STJ neutral position where the calcaneal bisection is everted relative to the longitudinal bisection of the distal one-third of the leg* (Fig. 8.6).

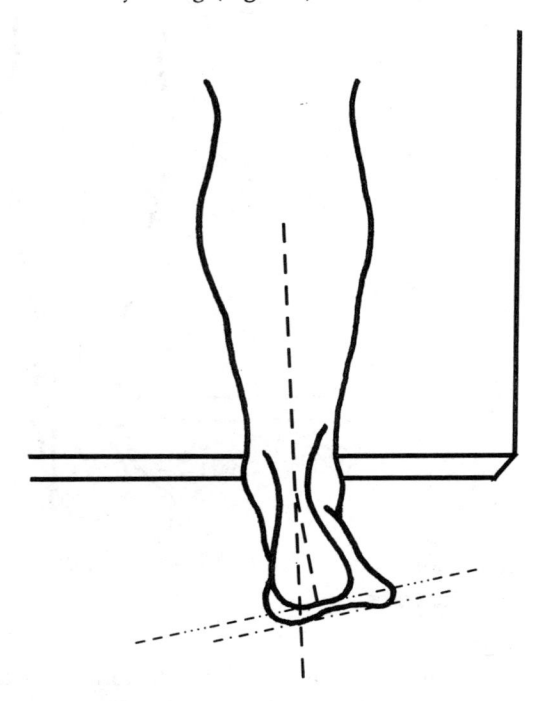

Figure 8.6.
Subtalar valgus.

8-20
If subtalar valgus is defined as a STJ neutral position where the calcaneal bisection is _____ to the leg bisector, one could reasonably infer that *subtalar varus is defined as a STJ neutral position in which the calcaneal bisection is* _____ *relative to the longitudinal bisection of the distal one-third of the leg* (Fig. 8.7).

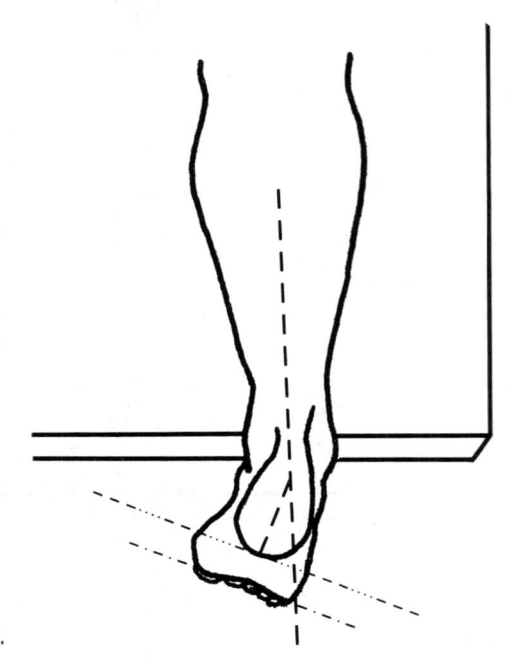

Figure 8.7.
Subtalar varus.

everted, inverted

8-21
Clinically, we see a much greater number of cases in which the calcaneus is inverted relative to the distal one-third the leg—i.e., subtalar _____.

8: FACTORS AFFECTING REARFOOT POSITION

varus

8-22
There are three main etiologic factors which are considered for subtalar varus (Fig. 8.8).

A varus torsion in either the talus or in the calcaneus itself can cause subtalar varus.

Also, a relative varus position of the distal tibial epiphysis can result in subtalar _____.

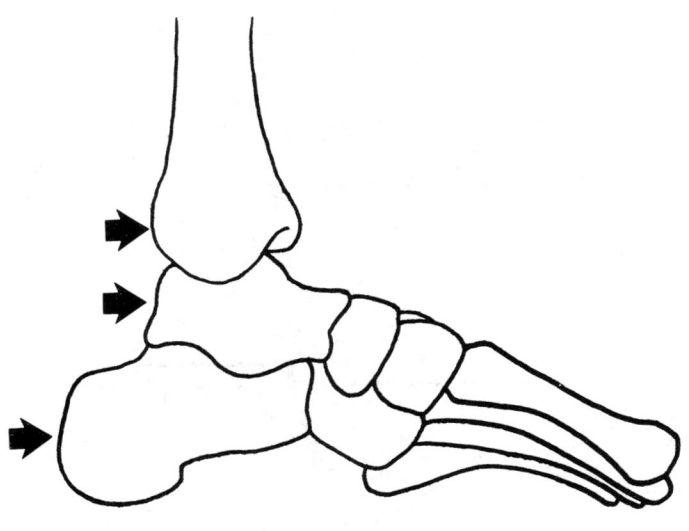

Figure 8.8.
Subtalar varus can be caused by abnormalities in the distal tibial epiphysis, the talus, and/or the calcaneus.

varus

8-23
Subtalar valgus, an _____ position of the calcaneus relative to the distal one-third of the leg, has similar etiologic factors as does subtalar varus.

That is to say, a valgus in either the _____ or the _____ or a relative valgus position of the distal _____ _____ can all result in a subtalar valgus condition.

everted, talus, calcaneus, tibial epiphysis

8-24
A condition in which the calcaneal bisector is everted relative to the leg bisector is called subtalar _____ and is less common than subtalar _____.

valgus, varus

8-25
Note that the three main etiologies discussed for subtalar varus—varus torsion of the _____ or _____ or a relative varus position of the _____ _____ _____—will affect the relationship of the calcaneus to the distal leg.

As a result of this alteration, the position of the calcaneus (and, hence, the STJ) relative to the ground will also be changed.

talus, calcaneus, distal tibial epiphysis

8-26
If the calcaneus is inverted *relative to the ground* with the STJ in its neutral position, this is called *rearfoot varus* (Fig. 8.9A).

If the calcaneus is inverted relative to the distal one-third of the leg with the STJ neutral, this is called _____ _____ (Fig. 8.9B).

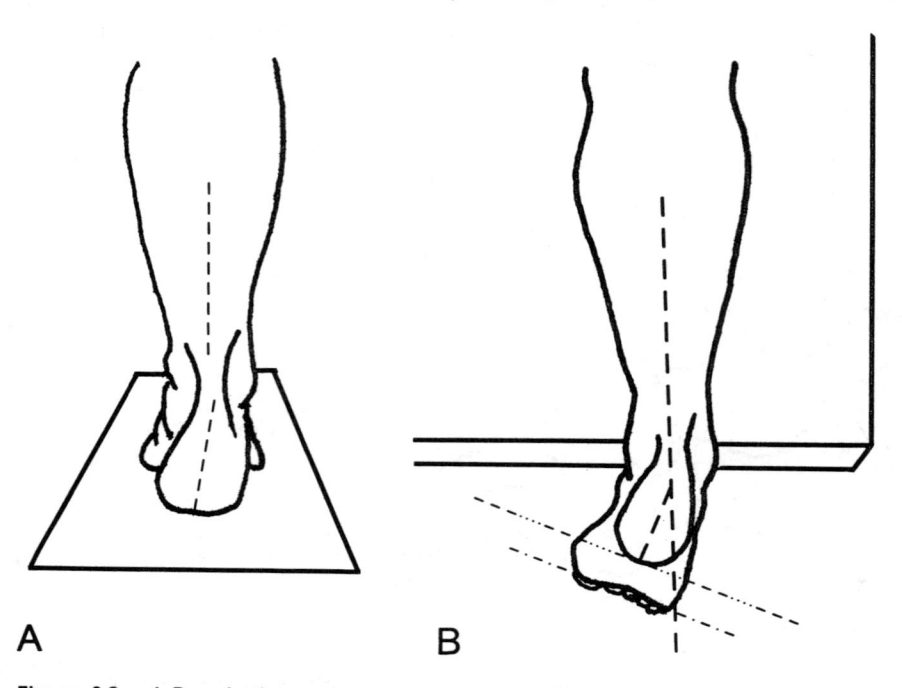

Figure 8.9. A, Rearfoot varus.

subtalar varus

8-27
When the calcaneus is inverted relative to the ground with the STJ neutral, i.e., _____ _____, all etiologies which could ultimately alter the position of the calcaneus to the ground must be considered.

Likewise, similar etiologies must be assessed when the calcaneus is *everted to the ground*, i.e., rearfoot _____.

rearfoot varus, valgus

8-28
Abnormalities which alter the position of the calcaneus to the ground could include those of subtalar varus and subtalar valgus or conditions which alter the normal frontal plane position of the tibia.

8-29
So, rearfoot varus could be caused by subtalar _____ or by an alteration of the normal _____ plane position of the tibia.

8: FACTORS AFFECTING REARFOOT POSITION

varus, frontal

8-30

Tibial varum is a condition in which the tibia is bowed toward the midline in the frontal plane, causing its distal aspect to be inverted relative to its proximal aspect. As a result, the normal frontal plane position of the tibia is altered (Fig. 8.10).

This condition, tibial varum, could then cause the calcaneus to be *(inverted/parallel/everted)* relative to the ground when the STJ is neutral, thus causing rearfoot _____.

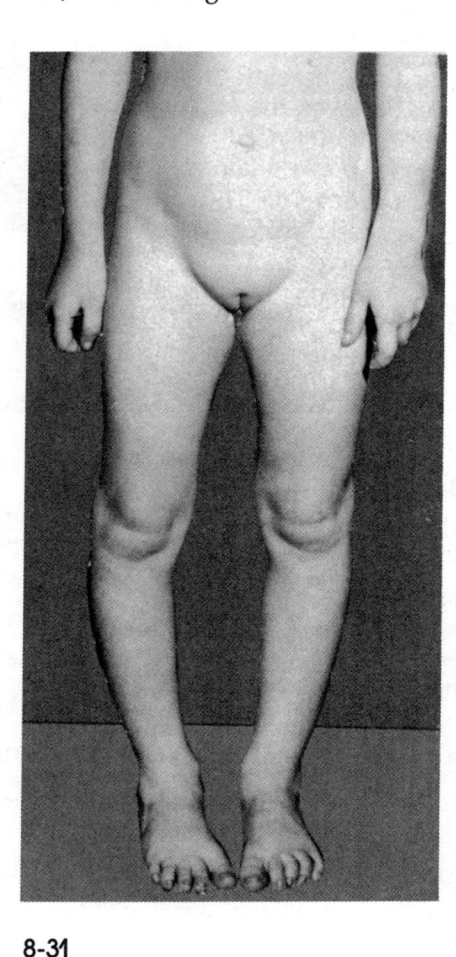

Figure 8.10. Tibial varum, secondary to Blount's disease. (Reproduced with permission from Salter RB: *Textbook of Disorders and Injuries of the Musculoskeletal System,* ed. 2. Baltimore, Williams & Wilkins, 1983, p 309.)

inverted, varus

8-31

The converse of tibial varum is tibial valgum, which is not frequently seen. However, mild degrees of tibial varum (1° to 4°) are seen commonly.

8-32

A condition which generally results in strong and persistent STJ pronation is called *tarsal coalition*.

A tarsal coalition can be defined as *an abnormal union between two (or more) tarsal bones* (Fig. 8.11).

Figure 8.11.
A calcaneonavicular tarsal coalition. (Reproduced with permission from Salter RB: *Textbook of Disorders and Injuries of the Musculoskeletal System,* ed. 2. Baltimore, Williams & Wilkins, 1983, p 121.)

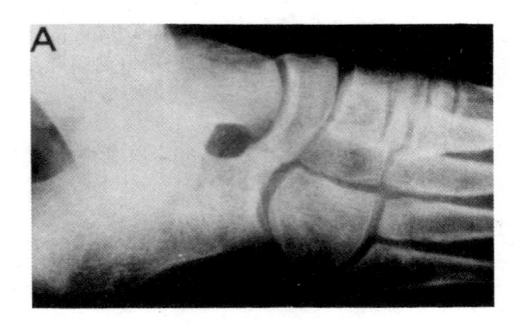

8-33

There are three types of tarsal coalition: syndesmosis, synchondrosis, and synostosis (respectively fibrous, cartilaginous, and bony unions).

Tarsal coalitions generally result in strong and persistent STJ _____.

8-34

pronation

In tarsal coalitions, because of the abnormal union between two _____ _____, *a restriction of STJ motion is an essential of diagnosis.*

8-35

tarsal bones

While there is no irritation of the STJ with a synostosis (bony union), there is usually significant irritation of the articular surfaces with a syndesmosis or synchondrosis.

This irritation occurs because the body tries to get more motion out of the STJ than the abnormal union of tarsal bones will allow.

The compensation that one will usually see clinically is strong and _____ STJ pronation.

8-36

persistent

The STJ pronation in a patient with tarsal coalition will last throughout the entire gait cycle—i.e., through both the stance and _____ phases of gait.

8: FACTORS AFFECTING REARFOOT POSITION

swing

8-37
The reason that chronic pronation is present in patients with syndesmosis and synchondrosis (respectively _____ and _____ unions) is that by keeping the STJ maximally pronated, STJ motion and, hence, irritation is limited.

fibrous, cartilaginous, restriction

Recall that an essential of diagnosis for tarsal coalition is a _____ of STJ motion.

8-38
To review, rearfoot varus denotes an (*inverted/parallel/everted*) position of the _____ relative to the _____ when the STJ is in its neutral position.

inverted, calcaneus, ground

8-39
Some etiologies of rearfoot varus are the same as those of _____ varus.

subtalar

8-40
Other etiologies of rearfoot varus include conditions which alter the normal _____ plane orientation of the _____.

frontal, tibia

8-41
Rearfoot valgus is a condition in which the calcaneus is _____ to the _____ when the STJ is in its neutral position.

everted, ground

8-42
The etiologic factors of rearfoot valgus include those of _____ _____, namely a valgus torsion of the _____ or _____. Additionally, a relative valgus position of the distal _____ _____ can also cause rearfoot valgus.

subtalar valgus, talus, calcaneus, tibial epiphysis

8-43
One condition in which the distal aspect of the tibia is inverted relative to its proximal aspect is called _____ _____.

tibial varum

8-44
Subtalar varus denotes a condition in which the _____ is (*inverted/parallel/everted*) relative to the distal _____-_____ of the leg with the STJ in its neutral position.

calcaneus, inverted, one-third

8-45
If a patient has tibial varum, would rearfoot varus also exist?

yes

8-46
This is because when the tibia is abnormally inverted, everything distal to it will also be abnormally inverted.

8-47
If a patient has tibial varum, would subtalar varus also exist?

no	**8-48** The reason for this is that while tibial varum alters the position of the calcaneus relative to the ground, it does *not* alter the relationship of the calcaneus to the distal _____-_____ of the _____. While subtalar varus may occur concomitantly with tibial varum, it is not a result of tibial varum.
one-third, leg	**8-49** Tarsal coalition, an abnormal union between two (or more) tarsal bones, is a condition which results in strong and persistent _____ _____.
STJ pronation	**8-50** While there is usually not motion (and, therefore, irritation) with a synostosis (i.e., a _____ union), there usually is irritation with a _____ or _____.
bony, syndesmosis, synchondrosis	**8-51** The body tries to stop the irritation about the joint by maintaining the STJ in a maximally _____ position.
pronated	**8-52** An essential of diagnosis of tarsal coalition is a _____ of STJ motion.
restriction	**8-53** Clinically, subtalar varus (and valgus) and rearfoot varus (and valgus) are used almost exclusively to define neutral rearfoot position. While abnormal muscle function may alter rearfoot relationships, osseous abnormalities (excluding tarsal coalitions) are the most common etiologies for altered rearfoot position. This ends the chapter. The following two chapters will deal with specific measurements of STJ parameters and how to interpret them.

Questions

1. Any muscular dysfunction which alters the balance between pronators and supinators of the STJ has the capacity to affect rearfoot position.
   a. true
   b. false

FRAME 8-2

8: FACTORS AFFECTING REARFOOT POSITION   95

2. Which of the following are *supinators* of the STJ?

    a. anterior tibial
    b. posterior tibial
    c. short digital flexors
    d. a and b
FRAME 8-5   e. b and c

3. Which of the following is the *strongest pronator* of the STJ?

    a. extensor digitorum longus
    b. extensor digitorum brevis
    c. peroneus longus
    d. peroneus brevis
FRAME 8-14   e. peroneus tertius

4. Which of the following are etiologic factors for subtalar varus?

    a. varus torsion of the talus
    b. varus torsion of the calcaneus
    c. relative varus position of the distal tibial epiphysis
    d. a and b
FRAME 8-22   e. a, b, and c

5. A STJ neutral position in which the calcaneal bisection is *everted* relative to the longitudinal bisection of the distal one-third of the leg defines:

    a. rearfoot varus
    b. rearfoot valgus
    c. subtalar varus
    d. subtalar valgus
FRAME 8-19   e. tibial varum

6. When the STJ is in its neutral position and the calcaneus is inverted *relative to the ground*, this is called:

    a. rearfoot varus
    b. rearfoot valgus
    c. subtalar varus
    d. subtalar valgus
FRAME 8-26   e. tibial varum

7. A tarsal coalition:

    a. is an abnormal union between two (or more) tarsal bones
    b. results in strong and persistent STJ pronation
    c. does not cause a restriction of STJ motion
    d. a and b
FRAMES 8-32 and 8-34   e. a, b, and c

8. Which of the following are possible etiologic factors for rearfoot varus?

    a. varus torsion of the calcaneus
    b. varus torsion of the talus
    c. tibial varum
    d. a and b
FRAMES 8-28–8-30   e. a, b, and c

FRAME 8-30

9. *Tibial varum* is defined as a condition in which the tibia is bowed toward the midline in the transverse plane, causing its distal aspect to be inverted relative to its proximal aspect.
   a. true
   b. false

FRAMES 8-39–8-42

10. If a patient has tibial varum, would rearfoot varus *and* subtalar varus exist also?
    a. yes
    b. no

Answers

1. a
2. d
3. d
4. e
5. d
6. a
7. d
8. e
9. b
10. b

CHAPTER 9

Rearfoot and Subtalar Joint: Closed Kinetic Chain Measurement and Evaluation

- STJ review
- angle and base of gait
- neutral calcaneal stance position—measurement and interpretation
- relaxed calcaneal stance position—measurement and interpretation
- rearfoot varus and its compensatory mechanism
- rearfoot valgus and its compensatory mechanism
- effect of tibial varum on the rearfoot

9-1
Before we begin discussing the CKC STJ measurements and what they might mean, let's review some important points from previous chapters.

9-2
The axis of the STJ (Fig. 9.1) runs from dorsal, _____, and _____ to plantar, _____, and _____.

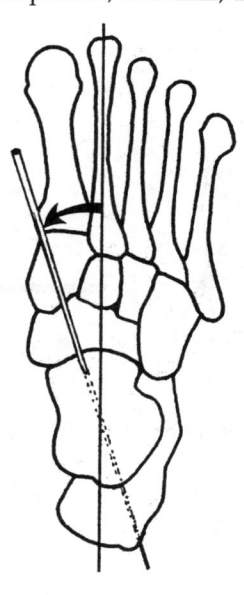

Figure 9.1.
A dorsal view of the STJ axis.

medial, distal, lateral, proximal	**9-3** It is angulated _____° from the _____ plane and _____° from the _____ plane.
42, transverse, 16, sagittal	**9-4** The muscles which pronate the STJ run (*medial/lateral*) to its axis.
lateral	**9-5** Conversely, the muscles which run medial to the STJ's axis cause _____ of the STJ to occur.
supination	**9-6** The muscles of the posterior leg, which are supinators of the STJ, run medial to the STJ. They are specifically the gastrocnemius and _____, the long _____ _____, and the _____ _____.
soleus, digital flexors, posterior tibial	**9-7** The muscle of the anterior leg which will supinate the STJ is the _____ _____.
anterior tibial	**9-8** The pronators of the STJ run _____ to the STJ axis. Specifically, they are the _____ longus, tertius, brevis, and the _____ _____.
lateral, peroneus, extensor digitorum longus	**9-9** The STJ's neutral position defines the point in its ROM from which there is _____ the amount of supination as there is pronation (Fig. 9.2).

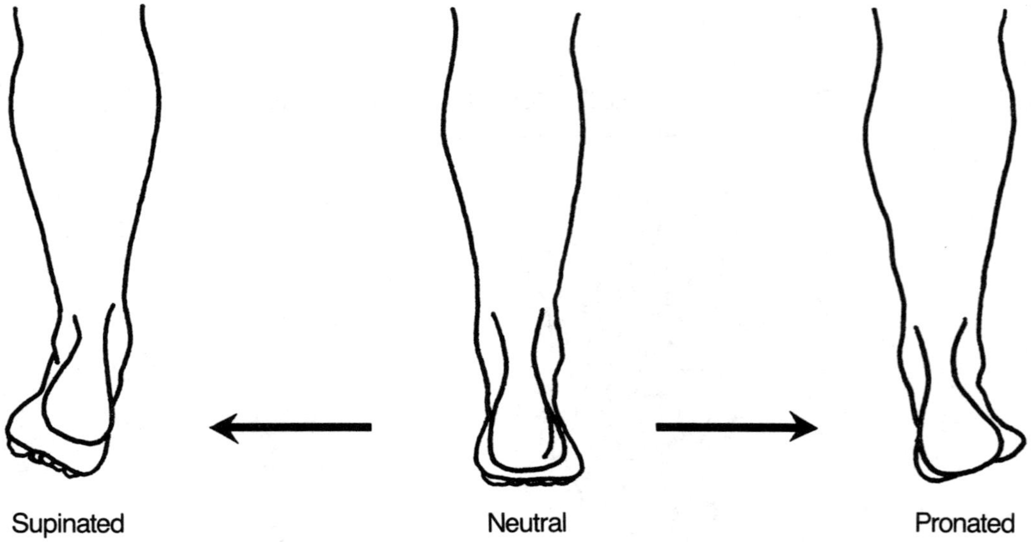

Supinated ← Neutral → Pronated

Figure 9.2. The STJ neutral position (NP) is found between the pronated and supinated positions.

twice	**9-10** When the normal STJ is in its neutral position, the calcaneus should be (*inverted/parallel/everted*) to the posterior bisection of the leg.
parallel	**9-11** If the calcaneus was inverted relative to the *leg* with the STJ neutral (Fig. 9.3), the condition would be called (*rearfoot/subtalar*) (*varus/valgus*).

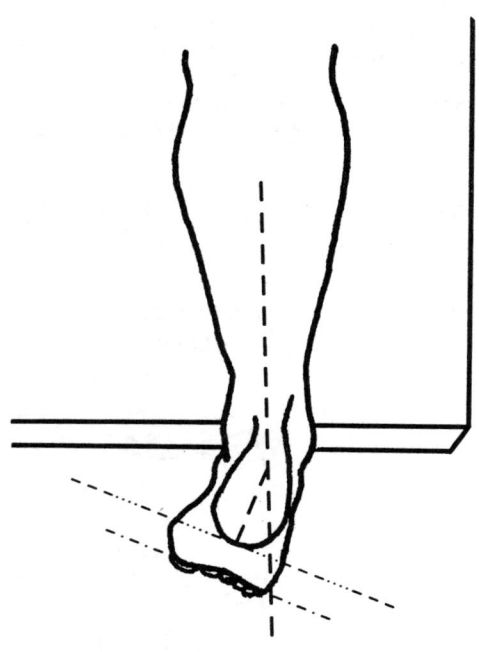

Figure 9.3.

subtalar varus	**9-12** If the calcaneus was inverted relative to the *ground* when the STJ was neutral (Fig. 9.4), the condition would be called _____ _____.

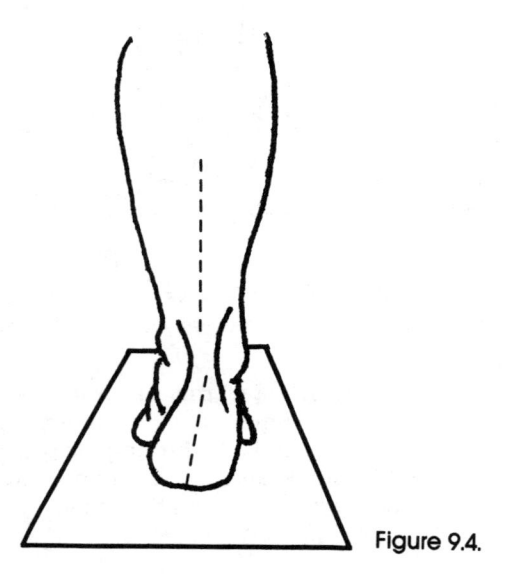

Figure 9.4.

rearfoot varus	**9-13** It would be reasonable to say that subtalar varus would be diagnosed after (*CKC/OKC*) STJ measurements.
OKC	**9-14** An example of a diagnosis that would be arrived at after evaluating CKC measurements is _____ varus.
rearfoot	**9-15** Anything proximal to the calcaneus can affect its position relative to the ground. A condition in which the distal aspect of the tibia is inverted relative to its proximal aspect is called _____ _____.
tibial varum	**9-16** Tibial varum (Fig. 9.5) is an abnormal frontal plane orientation of the tibia secondary to bowing in the _____ plane. (Tibial valgum—an everted position of the distal aspect of the tibia relative to its proximal aspect—is a rare clinical observation, and, hence, its discussion will be confined only to its definition.)

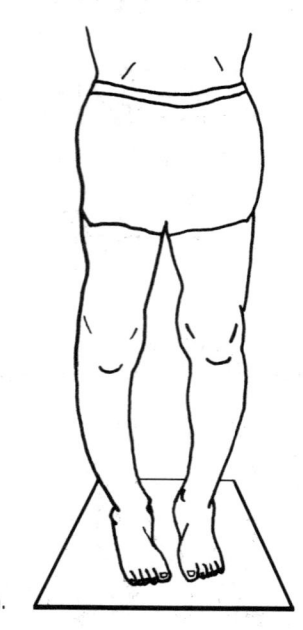

Figure 9.5. Tibial varum.

frontal	**9-17** Before discussing CKC lower extremity measurements in detail, some standard parameters of clinical measurement need to be explained. *Angle and base of gait* are terms which are frequently encountered clinically. The feet assume somewhat different positions depending on how the patient stands. By putting the patient in these *standard positions,* i.e., the angle and _____ of gait, we can *reproduce* measurements regardless of who sees the patient or when the patient is seen.

9: REARFOOT AND SUBTALAR JOINT: CLOSED KINETIC CHAIN MEASUREMENT AND EVALUATION

base

9-18
The *angle of gait* denotes the angle which the feet assume relative to the body's line of progression during gait. The angle of gait is estimated from observation of the patient's feet during several linear strides.

The *base of gait* refers to the closest width between the malleoli during the midstance period of gait. The base of gait is usually observed as one ankle passes the other.

By specifying a patient's _____ and _____ of gait, we are able to _____ measurements from one time and doctor to the next.

(An alternate method is to have the patient walk in place for 30 seconds and observe the position of the feet. By using this method, however, there is an increased apparent base of gait because the patient must widen their stance to support a stationary position.)

angle, base, reproduce

9-19
The shortest distance between a patient's malleoli during the midstance period of gait is called the _____ _____.

base of gait

9-20
The angle of gait is defined as the angulation of the feet from the patient's line of _____.

progression

9-21
The *neutral calcaneal stance position* is a CKC measurement—the angular relationship of the calcaneus to the ground with the STJ in its neutral position—then while the patient stands in their angle and base of gait.

9-22
So, to determine if a patient has, for example, rearfoot varus, one would need to assess the (*CKC/OKC*) measurement of the neutral _____ _____ _____.

9-23
Although we will not state it each time, note that *all weightbearing (CKC) measurements of the lower extremity are taken with the patient in the angle and base of gait.*

CKC, calcaneal stance position

9-24
A frontal plane deviation of the tibia in which the distal aspect is inverted relative to the proximal aspect is called _____ _____.

tibial varum

9-25
Likewise, if the tibia's distal aspect is everted relative to its proximal aspect, it is called tibial _____.

valgum

9-26
The angular relationship of the calcaneus to the ground with the STJ in its neutral position is called the _____ _____ _____ _____.

neutral calcaneal stance position

9-27
When the calcaneus is inverted relative to the ground in the neutral calcaneal stance position (*NCSP*) (Fig. 9.6), this condition is called _____ _____.

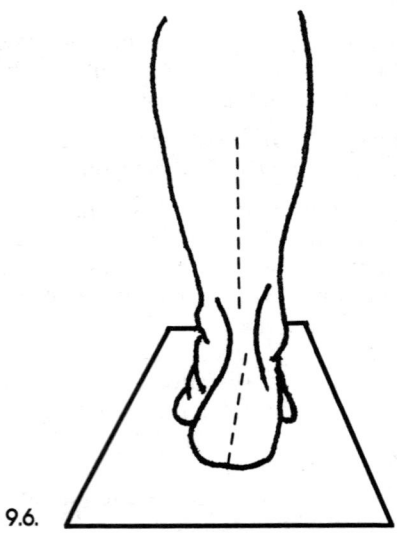

Figure 9.6.

rearfoot varus

9-28
Similarly, if the calcaneus was observed to be *everted* relative to the ground in the NCSP (Fig. 9.7), this would be called rearfoot _____.

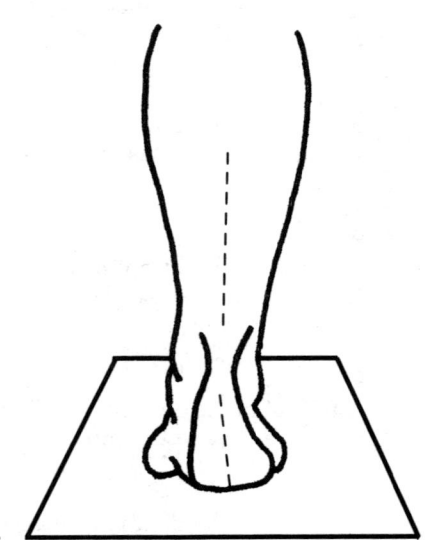

Figure 9.7.

9: REARFOOT AND SUBTALAR JOINT: CLOSED KINETIC CHAIN MEASUREMENT AND EVALUATION

valgus

9-29
Here's the clinical problem that will test your conceptual understanding.

A patient is observed to have a normal STJ neutral position (i.e., the calcaneus is parallel with the posterior bisection of the distal one-third of the leg when the STJ is in its neutral position).

On weightbearing, the patient is observed to have a 3° tibial varum.

The NCSP of this patient would be expected to be (*inverted/parallel/everted*) to the ground.

inverted

9-30
Thus, this patient would have a rearfoot _____.

varus

9-31
Remember, the STJ can have a normal neutral position relative to the leg, but if there is an abnormality proximally, it can affect the STJ's weightbearing position as indexed by the NCSP.

9-32
We measure tibial varum by quantitating the amount of frontal plane deviation of the distal tibia relative to a perpendicular to the ground.

Clinically, this is done by having the patient bear weight (in the angle and base of gait) and then placing the patient in the STJ neutral position (i.e., the _____ _____ _____ _____). A bisection is then placed over the posterior portion of the distal one-third of the leg.

A standard goniometer or a gravity goniometer is then used to determine how many degrees of tibial frontal plane deviation exist.

Clinically, it is common to see 1° or 2° of tibial varum. As mentioned earlier, tibial valgum is relatively rare.

neutral calcaneal stance position

9-33
The NCSP is measured with the patient standing in the angle and base of gait and with the STJ in its _____ position.

neutral

9-34
A similar measurement is taken with the patient standing *relaxed* in the angle and base of gait. The angular relationship *between the calcaneus and the ground* is determined.

This is known as the *relaxed calcaneal stance position*.

9-35
The position of the calcaneus relative to the ground with the patient standing relaxed in the angle and base of gait is called the _____ _____ _____ _____.

relaxed calcaneal stance position

9-36
In a patient with ideally normal values (i.e., no tibial varum and no subtalar varus/valgus), the neutral calcaneal stance position will be the same as the relaxed calcaneal stance position.

9-37
The relaxed calcaneal stance position (*RCSP*) varies from the NCSP when rearfoot varus is present.

9-38
If there is adequate pronatory motion available from the NCSP in a patient with rearfoot varus, the calcaneus will evert to the perpendicular. (This occurs so that the forces across the heel and forefoot may better be equilibrated.)

So, in a patient with rearfoot varus, the NCSP will show the calcaneus to be (*inverted/perpendicular/everted*) to the ground while the RCSP will show the calcaneus to be (*inverted/perpendicular/everted*) to the ground.

inverted, perpendicular

9-39
Rearfoot varus is classified as *compensated* when the calcaneus can evert to the perpendicular.

9-40
Can a patient with a NCSP in which the calcaneus is perpendicular to the ground have compensated rearfoot varus?

no

9-41
A diagnostic hallmark of rearfoot varus (Fig. 9.8) is an *inverted NCSP*.

If the NCSP is perpendicular to the ground, the RCSP will be (*inverted/perpendicular/everted*) to the ground.

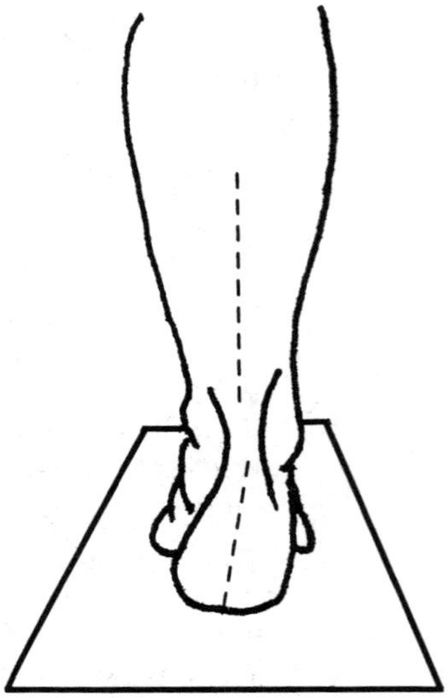

Figure 9.8.
A rearfoot varus foot in its NCSP.

perpendicular

9-42
If a patient's calcaneus is inverted to the ground in their NCSP and perpendicular to the ground in their RCSP, this would be called a _____ _____ _____.

compensated rearfoot varus

9-43
A diagnostic hallmark of rearfoot varus is a NCSP in which the calcaneus is _____ relative to the ground.

9: REARFOOT AND SUBTALAR JOINT: CLOSED KINETIC CHAIN MEASUREMENT AND EVALUATION

9-44
Rearfoot varus is classified as compensated when the calcaneus is (*inverted/perpendicular/everted*) to the ground with the STJ in the RCSP.

inverted

9-45
We call rearfoot varus *partially compensated* when, in the RCSP, the calcaneus is still inverted relative to the ground.

perpendicular

It is called partially compensated because the rearfoot varus deformity is not fully compensated by the calcaneus assuming a perpendicular relationship to the ground and thereby equilibrating forces on the _____ and _____.

9-46
If a patient is observed to have an inverted calcaneus in their NCSP and a less inverted calcaneus in their RCSP, they would be diagnosed as having a _____ _____ _____ _____.

heel, forefoot

9-47
Rearfoot valgus is defined by the calcaneus being _____ to the _____ when the STJ is in its _____ _____.

partially compensated rearfoot varus

9-48
Rearfoot valgus is not compensated for in the sense that rearfoot varus is. In rearfoot varus, the STJ pronates so that the forces of body weight may be equalized across the heel and forefoot.

everted, ground, neutral position

In a rearfoot valgus of greater than 2°, the body weight on the everted calcaneus will cause the STJ to pronate to the end of its ROM.

Rearfoot valgus may, however, be compensated by another deformity. For example, tibial varum would invert the calcaneus which would compensate for the everted position of rearfoot valgus (assuming that the degrees of both deformities were the same).

9-49
A rearfoot valgus of 3° would cause the STJ to maximally _____.

9-50
A rearfoot valgus of less than 2° does not change the STJ position from the NCSP.

pronate

9-51
If greater than 10° of rearfoot valgus exists, the head of the talus will usually contact the ground *before* the STJ completely pronates.

While this produces a severe flatfoot, the STJ is not pronated to the end of its ROM. This type of flatfoot is usually asymptomatic because the STJ does not reach the end of its pronatory ROM.

9-52
If a patient has a rearfoot valgus of less than 2°, does the STJ change its position from the NCSP?

9-53
If a patient has a rearfoot valgus of 3° to 10°, what happens to the STJ from the NCSP?

no

It maximally pronates.

9-54
Does the STJ maximally pronate if the rearfoot valgus is over 10°?

no

9-55
The STJ does not maximally pronate if rearfoot valgus exceeds 10° because STJ pronation is stopped by the head of the _____ contacting the ground.

talus

9-56
In fact, if the rearfoot valgus exceeds 10°, the RCSP is only 0° to 3° everted from the NCSP because the head of the talus contacts the _____ before the STJ can maximally pronate.

ground

9-57
So, if a patient had 12° of rearfoot valgus, their NCSP would be _____° everted, and their RCSP would be between _____° and _____° everted.

12, 12, 15

9-58
A deformity which causes the STJ to pronate to the perpendicular (if the pronatory ROM is available) is _____ _____.

rearfoot varus

9-59
A deformity which causes the STJ to pronate maximally (if the deformity is 3° to 10°) is _____ _____.

rearfoot valgus

9-60
To review, tibial varum is observed with a (CKC/OKC) measurement.

CKC

9-61
To measure for tibial varum, the patient is placed in the _____ and _____ of gait with both STJs in the _____ _____ stance position.

angle, base, neutral calcaneal

9-62
True or false: Both the NCSP and the RCSP are measured with the patient in the angle and base of gait.

true

9-63
True or false: To assess tibial varum, the patient must stand in the angle and base of gait with the STJ in the RCSP.

false

9-64
Tibial varum is assessed with the patient in the angle and base of gait, with the STJ in the NCSP. So, the statement in frame 9-46 would be false unless the RCSP was the same as the NCSP (which is unusual).

9-65
This completes the chapter.

The following chapter is a miniworkbook which lets you use calculations to illustrate and further understand the material concerning the STJ.

Questions

FRAME 9-14

1. Diagnosing rearfoot varus requires an *OKC* evaluation.
   a. true
   b. false

FRAME 9-23

2. All weightbearing measurements of the lower extremity are taken with the patient in the angle and base of gait.
   a. true
   b. false

FRAMES 9-28 AND 9-29

3. A patient with a normal STJ neutral position and 3° of tibial varum will have:
   a. rearfoot varus
   b. rearfoot valgus
   c. rearfoot valgus and subtalar valgus
   d. rearfoot varus and subtalar varus
   e. subtalar varus

FRAME 9-31

4. Tibial varum is measured by quantitating the amount of frontal plane deviation of the distal tibia relative to:
   a. a line connecting the ASIS and the lateral malleolus
   b. a line which is parallel to the proximal aspect of the tibia
   c. a line which connects the middle of the ankle and the middle of the knee
   d. a line which is perpendicular to the ground
   e. a line which is perpendicular to the ASIS level

FRAMES 9-23 AND 9-31

5. Tibial varum is measured with the patient in the:
   a. angle of gait
   b. base of gait
   c. RCSP
   d. a and b
   e. a, b, and c

FRAME 9-35

6. In a patient with ideally normal values (i.e., no tibial varum and no subtalar varus or valgus), the NCSP should be the same as the RCSP.
   a. true
   b. false

FRAME 9-37

7. In a patient with rearfoot varus, the calcaneus will evert *past* the perpendicular if there is adequate STJ pronatory motion.
   a. true
   b. false

8. A diagnostic hallmark of rearfoot varus is:
    a. accompanying tibial varum
    b. an everted RCSP
    c. an everted NCSP
    d. an inverted RCSP
    e. an inverted NCSP

FRAME 9-40

9. In a patient with 12° of rearfoot valgus:
    a. the calcaneus inverts to the perpendicular
    b. the calcaneus inverts to the end of the STJ ROM
    c. the STJ pronates to the end of its ROM
    d. the STJ does not pronate to the end of its ROM
    e. none of the above are correct

FRAME 9-50

10. In a patient with 3° of rearfoot valgus, the STJ compensates by:
    a. inverting the calcaneus to the perpendicular
    b. everting the calcaneus to the perpendicular
    c. inverting the calcaneus to the end of the STJ ROM
    d. everting the calcaneus to the end of the STJ ROM
    e. 3° of rearfoot valgus is not enough to cause any compensation to occur

FRAME 9-47

Answers

1. b	4. d	7. b	10. d
2. a	5. d	8. e	
3. a	6. a	9. d	

CHAPTER
10

Miniworkbook: Subtalar Joint Case Histories (Calculations and Interpretations)

Introduction

This miniworkbook will give you a chance to work with the same types of measurements and calculations that are found in the clinical biomechanical examination. After each case history, there is room for you to perform the calculations. When first working with the figures, you may find it helpful to draw out a stick figure diagram of STJ motion and tibial position as I have done in the sample which precedes the case histories (Fig. 10.1).

The data that you will be given is the same as that which you would collect if you were performing the examination yourself. It includes the amount of inversion and eversion from a line parallel with the distal one-third of the leg. This will allow you to determine the STJ neutral position (NP) relative to the leg. Concomitantly, it will allow you to diagnose a subtalar deformity (as measured between calcaneus and leg) if one is present. Tibial varum/valgum will be included in the case histories as well so that you are able to determine the

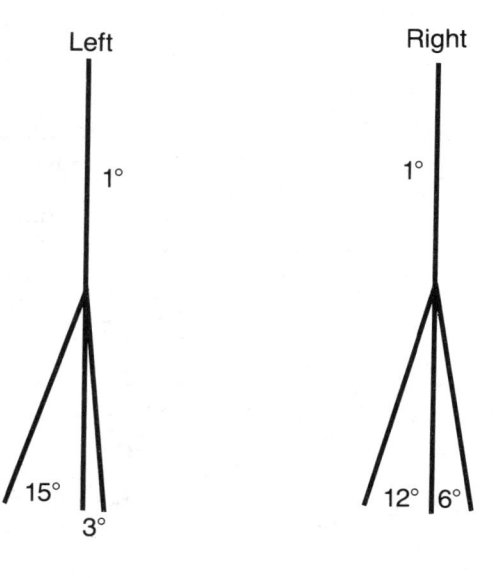

Figure 10.1.
A simple stick figure diagram may help to visualize some of the findings of a biomechanical examination.

NCSP and RCSP. By determining these two values, you will be able to diagnose rearfoot varus/valgus if it is present.

The symptomatology described is consistent with that which one may observe given the pathology presented. While these histories do not include all possible symptoms for a given pathologic state, they do help illustrate common symptom constellations which are seen clinically.

Following is an example which I have worked through to help get you started. At the end of the miniworkbook are the answers to each case history along with a brief discussion. If you have difficulty with the calculations and/or concepts, you may want to review the chapters germane to this material.

Sample Case History

Dr. S. C., a newly graduated dentist, comes into your office with a chief complaint of a "tired leg and foot only on my left side, usually occurring in the midafternoon, and getting worse as the day goes on."

While eliciting the history, you find out that Dr. C sees patients all day long and that he sits down only for lunch, walking and standing the rest of the time. After having dinner, he would like to go for an evening walk or jog, but his left foot and leg are too uncomfortable and fatigued to permit this.

He has noticed this fatigue only since being in practice. He admits that his ambulatory activity has increased substantially since he has started practice four months ago. His right side has been completely asymptomatic.

On examination, you find the following (Fig. 10.1):

	Right	Left
Maximum calcaneal inversion with STJ supination (relative to the distal one-third of the leg):	12	15
Maximum calcaneal eversion with STJ pronation (relative to the distal one-third of the leg):	6	3
Tibial varum:	1	1

Calculate the STJ NP, NCSP, RCSP.

Determine whether subtalar and/or rearfoot deformities exist and, if so, to what degree.

Calculations and Explanations

1. The STJ NP is determined by assessing the calcaneal position in maximum STJ supination and pronation relative to the posterior bisection of the distal one-third of the leg.

    The first step in this process is to find the total STJ ROM. This is done by adding the amount of inversion to the amount of eversion available to the calcaneus from a fixed point—i.e., a line parallel with the bisection of the posterior distal one-third of the leg.

    On the right side, adding 12 and 6, we get a total STJ ROM of 18°.

    On the left side, we also get 18° (15 + 3).

    We know that from the STJ NP there will be exactly two times as much supination as there is pronation available. Put another way, we know that with a total STJ ROM of 18°, there will be 12° of supination from the neutral position and 6° of pronation from the neutral position. (We divide the total STJ ROM into thirds. Then we assign two-thirds as supination and one-third as pronation.)

On the right (asymptomatic) side, we find that the STJ NP is on a line parallel with the posterior bisection of the distal one-third of the leg—i.e., essentially normal. Clinically, we would say that the STJ NP is 0° on the right side.

However, on the left (symptomatic) side, the point from which there is 12° of calcaneal inversion and 6° of calcaneal eversion is 3° inverted from the line which is parallel with the bisection of the posterior distal one-third of the leg. Clinically, we say that the left STJ NP is 3° inverted (the rest is understood).

So, the right STJ NP = 0°;
the left STJ NP = 3° inverted

2. Recall that subtalar deformity (i.e., subtalar varus or subtalar valgus) is defined by an abnormal relationship between the calcaneus and distal one-third of the leg.

Because the right STJ NP is neither inverted or everted from a line parallel with the posterior distal one-third of the leg, neither subtalar varus or subtalar valgus can be said to exist.

However, in Dr. C's symptomatic left side, the STJ NP is inverted relative to the distal one-third of the leg. Therefore, by definition, there exists a 3° subtalar varus condition on the left side (the STJ NP inverts the calcaneus to the leg by 3°).

So, the right STJ shows no subtalar deformity; the left STJ shows a 3° subtalar varus deformity.

3. To determine the NCSP (and whether or not a rearfoot deformity exists) and the RCSP, we need to consider the position of the calcaneus relative to the ground.

In order to properly assess these parameters, we need to consider the STJ NP, and also the position of the tibia, since an altered tibial position will alter the position of the STJ and calcaneus which are distal to it.

In Dr. C's case, we have measured 1° of tibial varum in both legs. This will then invert the calcaneus an additional 1° past where the STJ NP would put it.

In the right STJ, the NCSP would be 1° inverted (a 0° STJ NP plus 1° of tibial varum).

In the left STJ, the NCSP would be 4° inverted (a 3° inverted STJ NP plus 1° of tibial varum).

In both of this patient's lower extremities, the NCSP is inverted (i.e., the calcaneus is inverted relative to the ground when the STJ is in its NP). Therefore, by definition, this patient has a rearfoot varus of 1° on the right and 4° on the left.

Recall that if a patient has a rearfoot varus, he will compensate by bringing the calcaneus to a position perpendicular to the ground so that weight is more evenly distributed across the forefoot and the heel. Therefore, Dr. C's RCSP would be 0° (i.e., the calcaneus is perpendicular to the ground) on both the right and left sides.

So, on the right—NCSP = 1° inverted, there is a 1° rearfoot varus, and the RCSP = 0°.

On the left side, NCSP = 4° inverted, there is a 4° rearfoot varus, and the RCSP = 0°.

Dr. C. was probably symptomatic on the left side because he was having to pronate his STJ excessively to compensate for the 4° rearfoot varus (he's using a full two-thirds [4°] of his pronatory ROM to get the calcaneus perpendicular to the ground). As will be explained in Chapter 11, pronation makes the muscles of the foot and leg work much harder to provide stability. The reason for this is that instead of acting on a relatively stable structure (as the foot is when the STJ is at its NP), the muscles are acting on a much less stable structure (remember the pronated foot is a "loose bag of bones"). Because the foot is less stable, the muscles have to work that much harder to keep it stable. This is why patients with chronic excessive pronation frequently experience fatigue in the overworked musculature.

In this example, I have tried to give an idea of not only the calculations but the reasoning behind them as well. It is imperative that the clinical findings be conceptualized in this manner in order to fully understand the pathologic states. This will become even more important later when the effects of pathology on gait and the effects of multiple simultaneous deformities are discussed.

The material in this miniworkbook is not extremely difficult, but it may take some practice working with the figures and concepts before fluency is achieved. Don't forget: Drawing stick figures may help out when you are first getting started.

Case History #1

Ms. G. B., a 34-year-old jogger, presents to your office with a chief complaint of "leg fatigue and pain on the inside of my knees after I jog."

Ms. B.'s history reveals that she has only experienced these symptoms since she began jogging five months ago. The jogging terrain is dirt paths and grass. She does the appropriate stretching exercises for 10 minutes before and after jogging. The fatigue and knee pain are noticeable about one-half mile into the run, which usually is about one and one-half miles long, three to four times a week in the early mornings. She has not timed her runs, but other runners pass her frequently; she hardly passes others at all.

When she started, the knee pain and fatigue were usually gone by the next day. During the last month or two, the fatigue is still gone by the next day, but the knee pain has been generally persistent and seems to have worsened. While the knee pain is still not keeping her from jogging, she is still experiencing extreme discomfort and is concerned about what is going on.

On examination, you find the following:

	Right	Left
Maximum calcaneal inversion with STJ supination (relative to the distal part of the leg):	20	19
Maximum calcaneal eversion with STJ pronation (relative to the distal part of the leg):	4	5
Tibial varum:	4	3

Calculate the STJ NP, NCSP, and RCSP.

Determine whether subtalar and/or rearfoot deformities exist and, if so, to what degree. If rearfoot varus exists, determine if it is fully or partially compensated.

Case History #2

Mrs. V. H., a 59-year-old housewife, presents to you with a chief complaint of a "bunion that hurts on my left foot."

Her history reveals that the bunion has been slowly progressive over a period of many years. She first noticed it when she was in her late twenties.

She fractured her right leg when she was seven, after being thrown from a horse. With questioning, she does relate some "tiredness" in both legs after washing the dishes at night.

On examination, you find the following:

	Right	Left
Maximum calcaneal inversion with STJ supination (relative to the distal one-third of the leg):	15	17
Maximum calcaneal eversion with STJ pronation (relative to the distal one-third of the leg):	6	4
Tibial varum:	1	2

Calculate the STJ NP, NCSP, and RCSP.

Determine whether subtalar and/or rearfoot deformities exist and, if so, to what degree. If rearfoot varus exists, determine if it is fully or partially compensated.

Case History #3

Ms. O. M., a 27-year-old calligrapher, presents with a chief complaint of "spraining my right ankle all the time."

Ms. M. relates that for "many years" she has had what are apparently inversion sprains of her right ankle. She does mention that the first time she sustained a sprain she was wearing high-heeled shoes at a dance. She relates no history of any other trauma.

On examination, you find the following:

	Right	Left
Maximum calcaneal inversion with STJ supination (relative to the distal one-third of the leg):	16	15
Maximum calcaneal eversion with STJ pronation (relative to the distal one-third of the leg):	2	3
Tibial varum:	3	2

Calculate the STJ NP, NCSP, and RCSP.

Determine whether subtalar and/or rearfoot deformities exist and, if so, to what degree. If rearfoot varus exists, determine if it is fully or partially compensated.

Case History #4

Mr. K. S., a 45-year-old contractor, presents to your office with a chief complaint of "fatigue in my feet after I've walked around the construction site a little bit."

On further questioning, Mr. S. relates that the fatigue comes on around mid-day and seems a little worse in the right foot. The remainder of the history is noncontributory.

On examination, you find the following:

	Right	Left
Maximum calcaneal inversion with STJ supination (relative to the distal one-third of the leg):	28	26
Maximum calcaneal eversion with STJ pronation (relative to the distal one-third of the leg):	2	7
Tibial varum:	4	4

Calculate the STJ NP, NCSP, and RCSP.

Determine whether subtalar and/or rearfoot deformities exist and, if so, to what degree. If rearfoot varus exists, determine if it is fully or partially compensated.

Case History #5

Mr. F. C., a 32-year-old road worker, presents to you with a chief complaint of "arch pain in both of my feet."

Historically, Mr. C. has had painful arches during most of his adult life. He has recently started to supervise at his job and walks much more than he did before. Along with this increase in ambulatory activity has come a significant increase in his level of discomfort.

On examination, you find the following:

	Right	Left
Maximum calcaneal inversion with STJ supination (relative to the distal one-third of the leg):	8	11
Maximum calcaneal eversion with STJ pronation (relative to the distal one-third of the leg):	10	10
Tibial varum:	1	0

Calculate the STJ NP, NCSP, and RCSP.

Determine whether subtalar and/or rearfoot deformities exist and, if so, to what degree. If rearfoot varus exists, determine if it is fully or partially compensated.

Case History #6

Ms. T. D., a 19-year-old tennis star, presents to you with a chief complaint of a painful "callus on the ball of my right foot."

While obtaining the history, you find out that Ms. D. has "always" had her callus. Since she started professional training eight months ago, which includes running five miles a day, she has noticed that it has gotten larger and more uncomfortable.

Before obtaining her STJ measurements, you notice that the callus is located under the second metatarsal head of the right foot. Additionally, she has a small bunion deformity on the right foot.

On examination, you find the following:

	Right	Left
Maximum calcaneal inversion with STJ supination (relative to the distal one-third of the leg):	14	13
Maximum calcaneal eversion with STJ pronation (relative to the distal one-third of the leg):	13	11
Tibial varum:	1	2

Calculate the STJ NP, NCSP, and RCSP.

Determine whether subtalar and/or rearfoot deformities exist and, if so, to what degree. If rearfoot varus exists, determine if it is fully or partially compensated.

Case History #7

Mr. L. K., a 48-year-old restauranteur, presents to you with a chief complaint of "a tired feeling in my feet and legs."

Mr. K. has had this for "several years" and is mostly on his feet from around 6 A.M. until 7 P.M. He has tried wearing various types of shoes but to no avail.

On examination, you find the following:

	Right	Left
Maximum calcaneal inversion with STJ supination (relative to the distal one-third of the leg):	20	19

	Right	Left
Maximum calcaneal eversion with STJ pronation (relative to the distal one-third of the leg):	13	11
Tibial varum:	3	1

Calculate the STJ NP, NCSP, and RCSP.

Determine whether subtalar and/or rearfoot deformities exist and, if so, to what degree. If rearfoot varus exists, determine if it is fully or partially compensated.

Case History #8

Mr. G. A., a 26-year-old jogger, presents to your office with a chief complaint of "painful calluses on the bottom of my right foot."

Mr. A. states that he has had this since his late teens but that it has built up faster and hurt more since he started jogging four months ago. He also relates a history of significant foot and leg pain, more on the right than the left, after walking a lot or jogging.

There is a history of a fractured leg after being thrown from a horse at the age of 12.

On examination, you find the following:

	Right	Left
Maximum calcaneal inversion with STJ supination (relative to the distal one-third of the leg):	15	15
Maximum calcaneal eversion with STJ pronation (relative to the distal one-third of the leg):	15	15
Tibial valgum:	0	6

Calculate the STJ NP, NCSP, and RCSP.

Determine whether subtalar and/or rearfoot deformities exist and, if so, to what degree. If rearfoot varus exists, determine if it is fully or partially compensated.

Case History #9

Ms. S. U., a 30-year-old pharmaceutical representative, presents to you with a chief complaint of "a painful bump on the back of my right foot."

Ms. U. has noticed this more since starting her present job nine months ago, however, she has been aware of it since her early twenties. She wears sensible shoes with a two-inch heel and a good heel counter.

On examination, you find the following:

	Right	Left
Maximum calcaneal inversion with STJ supination (relative to the distal one-third of the leg):	19	16
Maximum calcaneal eversion with STJ pronation (relative to the distal one-third of the leg):	5	11
Tibial varum:	3	3

Calculate the STJ NP, NCSP, and RCSP.

Determine whether subtalar and/or rearfoot deformities exist and, if so, to what degree. If rearfoot varus exists, determine if it is fully or partially compensated.

Case History #10

Mr. B. V., a 54-year-old vintner, presents to you with a chief complaint of "pain in my arches."

Historically, Mr. V. has experienced discomfort in his arches for "20 or 30 years." He had arch supports made for him many years ago which relieved his symptoms. When he was vacationing at Martha's Vineyard, he lost the supports; within a few days, he had significant discomfort.

On examination, you find the following:

	Right	Left
Maximum calcaneal inversion with STJ supination (relative to the distal one-third of the leg):	14	15
Maximum calcaneal eversion with STJ pronation (relative to the distal one-third of the leg):	7	6
Tibial varum:	4	3

Calculate the STJ NP, NCSP, and RCSP.

Determine whether subtalar and/or rearfoot deformities exist and, if so, to what degree. If rearfoot varus exists, determine if it is fully or partially compensated.

Case History #1

1. Right STJ NP = 4° inverted
   Left STJ NP = 3° inverted
   Remember, first obtain the total STJ ROM (24° on both sides). Realize that from the STJ NP, one-third of the motion will be pronatory and two-thirds will be supinatory.
2. Because the STJ NP is inverted (from the distal one-third of the leg), subtalar varus exists bilaterally.
   Right side = 4° subtalar varus
   Left side = 3° subtalar varus
3. Right NCSP = 8° inverted
   Left NCSP = 6° inverted
   Recall that the amount of tibial varum is additive with the amount of subtalar varus in determining where the calcaneus rests relative to the ground when the STJ is in its neutral position.
4. By definition, the right side has an 8° rearfoot varus deformity and the left side has a 6° rearfoot varus deformity.
   (Remember, rearfoot varus is defined by an inverted position of the calcaneus relative to the ground when the STJ is in its neutral position.)
5. Right RCSP = 0°
   Left RCSP = 0°
   Both STJs have enough pronatory motion available from the neutral position to allow the calcaneus to move perpendicular to the ground, thereby equalizing forces on the heel and forefoot.
6. Both sides are completely compensated rearfoot varus deformities because the calcaneus reaches the perpendicular on both sides.

DISCUSSION

Ms. B. is pronating completely to the end of her ROM in the right STJ and is using 6 of 8° of STJ pronatory motion to get her calcaneus perpendicular on the left. This excessive amount of pronation will easily cause the fatigue in her leg muscles that she has described. Sometimes, people will only notice the fatigue in their legs and not in their feet and vice versa. Other times, as in Dr. C.'s case, they will notice fatigue in both areas.

Remember, chronic pronation has fatigue in the legs and/or feet as one of its hallmarks. Some patients, like Ms. G. B., only appreciate the fatigue when the lower extremities are extremely stressed, as in jogging. Others, like Dr. S. C., feel the fatigue with only a slight amount of increased ambulatory activity.

The bilateral medial knee pain that Ms. G. B. described is not infrequently seen in runners with excessive pronation. Recall that with STJ pronation, there is internal rotation of the tibia. This stresses the medial collateral ligaments of the knee and causes pain as a result of the ensuing inflammation.

These types of symptoms frequently respond to limitation of the excessive pronation by orthotic devices.

Case History #2

1. Right STJ NP = 1° inverted
   Left STJ NP = 3° inverted
2. Right side = 1° subtalar varus
   Left side = 3° subtalar varus
3. Right NCSP = 2° inverted
   Left NCSP = 5° inverted
4. Right side = 2° rearfoot varus
   Left side = 5° rearfoot varus
5. Right RCSP = 0°
   Left RCSP = 0°
6. Both sides are completely compensated rearfoot varus deformities.

DISCUSSION

Mrs. H. has a substantial rearfoot varus on the left side which is also the side which has the symptomatic bunion. On this side, she is pronating significantly in order to bring her calcaneus to the perpendicular.

Recall that pronation effectively shortens the length of the side which is pronating. It is not unusual to see a limb length discrepancy in a patient who has sustained a leg fracture as a child. The limb which sustained the trauma is usually the shorter one. The contralateral side will pronate excessively in order to help equalize the length of the two limbs.

In Mrs. H.'s case, the side with the bunion deformity was the one which pronated excessively. Excessive pronation produces a malalignment of the flexor hallucis and flexor digitorum longus (and attached quadratus plantae) tendons. This alters the normal dynamic balance which exists about the first metatarsophalangeal joint and thereby causes a bunion formation in many situations. (It is not at all unusual to see associated hammertoes of the lesser digits for the same reasons.)

Case History #3

1. Right STJ NP = 4° inverted
   Left STJ NP = 3° inverted
2. Right side = 4° subtalar varus
   Left side = 3° subtalar varus
3. Right NCSP = 7° inverted
   Left NCSP = 5° inverted
4. Right side = 7° rearfoot varus
   Left side = 5° rearfoot varus
5. Right RCSP = 1° inverted
   Left RCSP = 0°

   Recall that from the STJ NP, there is only one-third of the total ROM available for pronation (in this case, 6 of 18 degrees). On the right side, the 6° of pronatory motion will only take the calcaneus to a 1° inverted position. On the left side, however, the 6° are more than enough to bring the calcaneus perpendicular to the ground.

6. Right side = partially compensated rearfoot varus
   Left side = completely compensated rearfoot varus

   The right side is only partially compensated because, even with maximum pronation, the calcaneus is still inverted to the ground.

DISCUSSION

Patients with partially compensated rearfoot varus can suffer chronic ankle sprains as a result of this condition. Since the calcaneus is always inverted, even when the STJ is maximally pronated, the force of the body weight is thrown more laterally through the ankle joint, thus predisposing to chronic inversion ankle sprains.

Note that Ms. M. suffered her first sprain while wearing high-heeled shoes. High heels cause the talus to be more plantarflexed than it is normally. This plantar flexion brings the narrower posterior portion of the talar dome into the ankle mortise. While the anterior part of the talar dome is thicker and allows almost no frontal plane motion at the ankle, the narrow posterior portion does not allow the same amount of stability. Thus, it is not unusual to see ankle sprains associated with the wearing of high-heeled shoes.

In this patient's case, the increased frontal plane motion at the ankle combined with the inverted position of the calcaneus and subsequent lateral displacement of the body weight through the ankle will strongly predispose to an inversion-type ankle sprain.

Case History #4

1. Right STJ NP = 8° inverted
   Left STJ NP = 4° inverted
2. Right side = 8° subtalar varus
   Left side = 4° subtalar varus
3. Right NCSP = 12° inverted
   Left NCSP = 8° inverted
4. Right side = 12° rearfoot varus
   Left side = 8° rearfoot varus
5. Right RCSP = 2° inverted
   Left RCSP = 0°
6. Right side = partially compensated rearfoot varus
   Left side = completely compensated rearfoot varus

DISCUSSION

On the right side, Mr. S. is pronating his STJ maximally and still not getting the calcaneus to the perpendicular. The right foot, therefore, is the most unstable that it can be. This would account for the greater appreciation of fatigue on the right side.

On the left side, the rearfoot varus is completely compensated. In fact, there is an additional 3° of pronatory motion available from the perpendicular. So, the patient is pronating excessively on the left side but not using up all of the pronatory motion. This makes the foot a little more stable than the one on the right. Because of this, the muscles of the right foot don't have to work quite as hard as their counterparts on the other foot, and, hence, the fatigue is less on the right side.

Note that in this example, there are two different STJ ROMs. While a patient's STJ ROMs are usually symmetrical, there may be small differences because of examiner's error or because they actually exist in a minority of patients.

Case History #5

1. Right STJ NP = 4° everted
   Left STJ NP = 3° everted
2. Right side = 4° subtalar valgus
   Left side = 3° subtalar valgus
3. Right NCSP = 3° everted
   Left NCSP = 3° everted

   The right NCSP is 3° everted instead of 4° because the tibial varum offsets the rearfoot valgus.

   The left NCSP is the same as the left STJ NP because no tibial varum exists on that side.
4. Right side = 3° rearfoot valgus
   Left side = 3° rearfoot valgus
5. Right RCSP = 9° everted
   Left RCSP = 10° everted

   The right RCSP is 9° everted because although the STJ fully pronates with a rearfoot valgus of over 2°, the tibial varum offsets the everted position by 1°. (If there had been no tibial varum on the right side, the RCSP would have been 10°.)

   The left RCSP is 10° because there is no tibial varum to offset the maximal STJ pronation that has occurred with the 3° rearfoot valgus.

DISCUSSION

In this example, both STJs are maximally pronating because of the rearfoot valgus in excess of 2°. Arch pain is a frequent complaint in patients whose STJ is forced to pronate to the end of its ROM with ambulatory activity.

CKC STJ pronation causes the arches of the feet to flatten, thus pulling the plantar fascia taut to a greater than normal degree. Inflammation of the plantar fascia ensues which is aggravated as more ambulation occurs. This explains how chronic plantar fasciitis of biomechanical etiology can be exacerbated with excessive STJ pronation during ambulatory activity.

Case History #6

1. Right STJ NP = 4° everted
   Left STJ NP = 3° everted
2. Right side = 4° subtalar valgus
   Left side = 3° subtalar valgus
3. Right NCSP = 3° everted
   Left NCSP = 1° everted

   (Remember: it is necessary to figure in how the tibial varum will change the calcaneal-to-ground relationship.)
4. Right side = 3° rearfoot valgus
   Left side = 1° rearfoot valgus
5. Right RCSP = 12° everted
   Left RCSP = 1° everted

   Recall that a rearfoot valgus deformity must be over 2° to cause the STJ to maximally pronate. If the rearfoot valgus deformity is 2° or less, the STJ will not be affected.

   (Another point worthy of consideration is that a foot with maximal STJ pronation will usually look like a flatfoot. This would certainly be the case with 12° of calcaneal eversion taking place.)

DISCUSSION

Because of the maximal pronation of the right foot, Ms. D. has developed a callus under the second metatarsal head. This occurs because the lateral side of the foot does not contact the ground with as much force as the medial side of the foot. (An everted rearfoot will tend to evert everything distal to it as well.) As will be discussed later, pronation of the STJ increases the ROM of the first ray, thereby making the second ray take the brunt of the force of body weight. Ms. D.'s recent increase in stressful ambulatory activity has evidently aggravated the existing situation.

It is important to point out that a callus under the second metatarsal head is a relatively infrequent sign of rearfoot valgus.

The bunion deformity that is in its early stages is a reflection of a chronic pronatory condition. If the excessive pronation can be limited during these early stages, there is a chance that the bunion deformity can be arrested or retarded in its development.

Case History #7

1. Right STJ NP = 2° everted
   Left STJ NP = 1° everted
2. Right side = 2° subtalar valgus
   Left side = 1° subtalar valgus
3. Right NCSP = 1° inverted
   Left NCSP = 0°

   The right NCSP is 1° inverted because of the tibial varum offsetting the everted position of subtalar valgus.

   Likewise, the left NCSP is 0° because the 1° of tibial varum cancels out the 1° of subtalar valgus.
4. Right side = 1° rearfoot varus
   Left side = calcaneus is perpendicular to the ground—i.e., no rearfoot varus or rearfoot valgus
5. Right RCSP = 0°
   Left RCSP = 0°

   The right RCSP is at 0° because of the compensatory mechanism for rearfoot varus (i.e., to bring the calcaneus perpendicular to the ground if adequate pronatory motion exists).

   The left RCSP is at 0° because the calcaneus stays perpendicular to the ground if no rearfoot varus or rearfoot valgus are present.
6. The right rearfoot varus is completely compensated.

DISCUSSION

The biomechanical status of Mr. K.'s feet is probably not the cause of his foot and leg fatigue. There is not any excessive pronation occurring on the left and only a very small amount occurring on the right.

Probably, this patient is having venous pooling in the absence of any useful pumping action by his leg muscles.

Case History #8

1. Right STJ NP = 5° everted
   Left STJ NP = 5° everted
2. Right side = 5° subtalar valgus
   Left side = 5° subtalar valgus
3. Right NCSP = 5° everted
   Left NCSP = 11° everted

   Remember: The NCSP is the result of not only the relation of the

STJ and calcaneus to the distal one-third of the leg but also the relationship of the distal one-third of the leg to the ground.

In this case, the left side has 6° of tibial valgum, i.e., an everted position of the distal aspect of the tibia. This does not offset the subtalar valgus (as does tibial varum) but instead adds to it. The result is a NCSP which is even more everted than the STJ NP.

In other words, there is even a larger degree of rearfoot valgus than there is of subtalar valgus because of the additional everting factor of tibial valgum.

4. Right side = 5° rearfoot valgus
   Left side = 11° rearfoot valgus
5. Right RCSP = 15° everted
   Left RCSP = 11° to 14° everted

Recall that when over 10° of rearfoot valgus exists, the head of the talus contacts the ground before all of the STJ pronatory motion is used up. Furthermore, the RCSP in these situations will be only 0° to 3° more than is the NCSP. In this case, it works out to between 11° and 14° everted for the RCSP on the left side.

Notice that in this case, the greater deformity is undergoing less abnormal compensatory pronation than the lesser deformity! This is usually the case when comparing a rearfoot valgus deformity of over 10° with one of 3° to 10°.

DISCUSSION

This case illustrates the apparently incongruous nature of the rearfoot valgus deformity. Rearfoot valgus of greater than 10° looks like a severe flatfoot deformity, however, there is less destructive force (i.e., STJ pronation) generated by the larger deformity than by the rearfoot valgus of 3° to 10°.

Evidently, judging by the asymmetry of the two tibia, Mr. A. may very well have acquired his 6° of tibial valgum after fracturing his leg as a boy. Usually, the tibia and joints of the feet are relatively symmetrical from one side to the other.

The callus on the bottom of the right foot is probably under the second metatarsal head—the most common location for a callus caused by rearfoot valgus. Recall from Case History #6 that rearfoot valgus alone does not frequently cause calluses to form. They do form when a lot of abnormal (pronatory) motion causes abnormal shearing forces to be generated under the metatarsal head. That is the situation in Mr. A.'s right foot (the one with the smaller degree of rearfoot valgus causing a greater amount of abnormal compensatory STJ pronation).

Case History #9

1. Right STJ NP = 3° inverted
   Left STJ NP = 2° everted
2. Right side = 3° subtalar varus
   Left side = 2° subtalar valgus
3. Right NCSP = 6° inverted
   Left NCSP = 1° inverted
4. Right side = 6° rearfoot varus
   Left side = 1° rearfoot varus
5. Right RCSP = 0°
   Left RCSP = 0°
6. Both sides are completely compensated rearfoot varus deformities.

DISCUSSION

The "painful bump" on the back of Ms. U.'s right foot is a retrocalcaneal prominence. These are frequently caused by shearing motion between the posterior superior surface of the calcaneus and the skin as the calcaneus moves during STJ pronation. The skin is held relatively immobile by the shoe counter and receives the brunt of the force rather than moving with the calcaneus and avoiding the insult.

Retrocalcaneal prominences develop when there is calcaneal motion with a heel counter providing frictional restraint.

Orthoses which diminish calcaneal eversion (i.e., STJ pronation) can significantly reduce the amount of friction generated at this area.

Case History #10

1. Right STJ NP = $0°$
   Left STJ NP = $1°$
2. Right side = no subtalar deformity
   Left side = $1°$ subtalar varus
3. Right NCSP = $4°$ inverted
   Left NCSP = $4°$ inverted
4. Right side = $4°$ rearfoot varus
   Left side = $4°$ rearfoot varus
5. Right RCSP = $0°$
   Left RCSP = $0°$
6. Both sides are completely compensated rearfoot varus deformities.

DISCUSSION

Mr. V. was having arch pain because of the STJ pronation necessary to completely compensate his rearfoot varus.

This case illustrates the importance of evaluating tibial varum or valgum, since no subtalar deformity was present on the right side.

Even though "arch supports" were made much differently from today's orthoses, diminution of abnormal compensatory STJ pronation was still achieved in varying degrees, albeit through a "hit or miss" approach. It is important in treatment of rearfoot (and forefoot) biomechanical pathology to prescribe orthoses which specifically address the problem which is present.

CHAPTER 11

Effects of Rearfoot Pathology on the Gait Cycle

- gait cycle review
- effects of STJ function during the gait cycle
- abnormal STJ pronation—effects locally and in the gait cycle
- hypermobility and its effects
- abnormal shearing forces and their effects
- rearfoot varus and equinus effects in the gait cycle
- rearfoot valgus and tarsal coalition effects in the gait cycle

11-1
Let's begin with a quick review of the gait cycle. The gait cycle is defined as that interval of time from heel strike of one foot to heel strike of the _____ foot at the next step.

same

11-2
The gait cycle is composed of weightbearing and non-weightbearing portions (Fig. 11.1), respectively the _____ phase and the _____ phase.

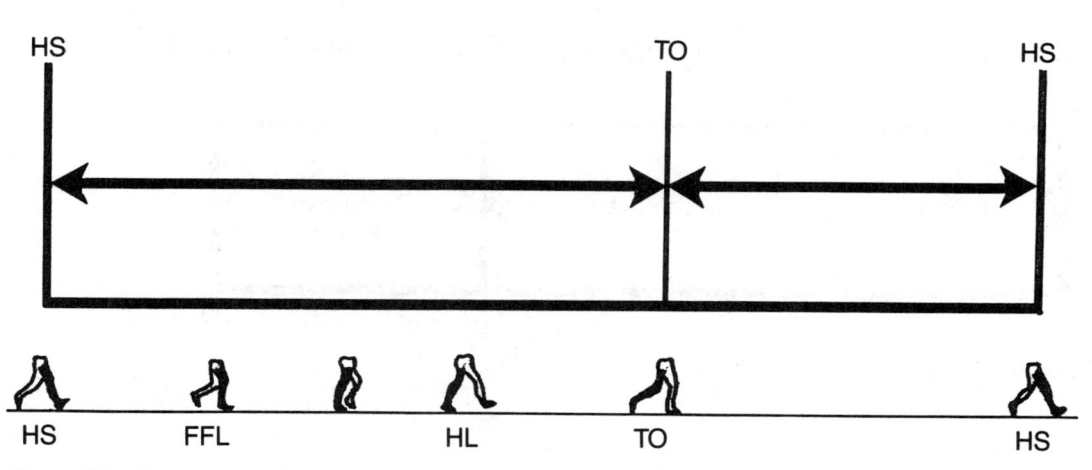

Figure 11.1. The complete gait cycle.

stance, swing	**11-3** The stance phase is divided into three major periods. In alphabetical order (and in order of their occurrence), they are the _____, _____, and _____ periods.
contact, midstance, propulsive	**11-4** The stance phase occurs between _____ _____ and _____ _____ of the same foot and occupies about 60% of the gait cycle.
heel strike, toe off	**11-5** The *contact period* of the stance phase occurs between _____ _____ of the same foot and _____ _____ of the opposite foot.
heel strike, toe off	**11-6** The midstance period starts just as the contact period ends, i.e., right after toe off of the _____ foot.
opposite	**11-7** The midstance period (which precedes the _____ period and comes after the _____ period) ends with heel lift of the same foot.
propulsive, contact	**11-8** To review, the contact period begins with _____ _____ of the _____ foot and ends with _____ _____ of the _____ foot.
heel strike, same, toe off, opposite	**11-9** The midstance period begins with _____ _____ of the _____ foot and ends with _____ _____ of the _____ foot.
toe off, opposite, heel lift, same	**11-10** The last period in the stance phase of gait is the _____ period.
propulsive	**11-11** The propulsive period begins with _____ _____ of the _____ foot and ends with _____ _____ of the _____ foot.
heel lift, same, toe off, same	**11-12** The stance phase of gait (Fig. 11.2) occupies roughly _____% of the gait cycle.

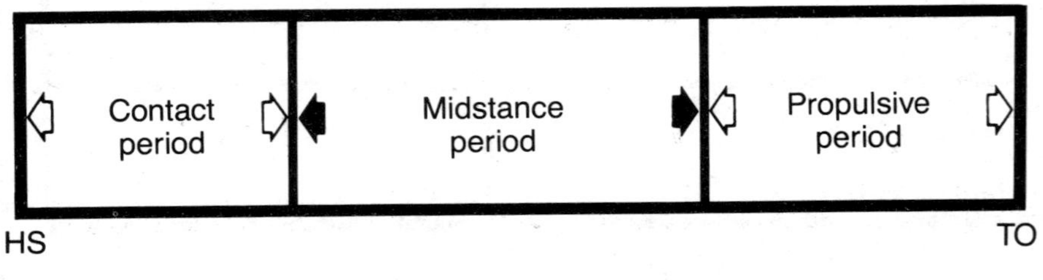

Contact period	Midstance period	Propulsive period

HS   TO

Figure 11.2. The stance phase of the gait cycle.

11: EFFECTS OF REARFOOT PATHOLOGY ON THE GAIT CYCLE

11-13
The non-weightbearing phase of the gait cycle is called the _____ phase and occupies the remaining _____% of the gait cycle.

60

11-14
The swing phase (Fig. 11.3) occurs between _____ _____ of the _____ foot and _____ _____ of the _____ foot.

swing, 40

```
|<--------- Stance phase --------->|<------ Swing phase ------>|
              60%                           40%
 HS                                HS                          TO
```

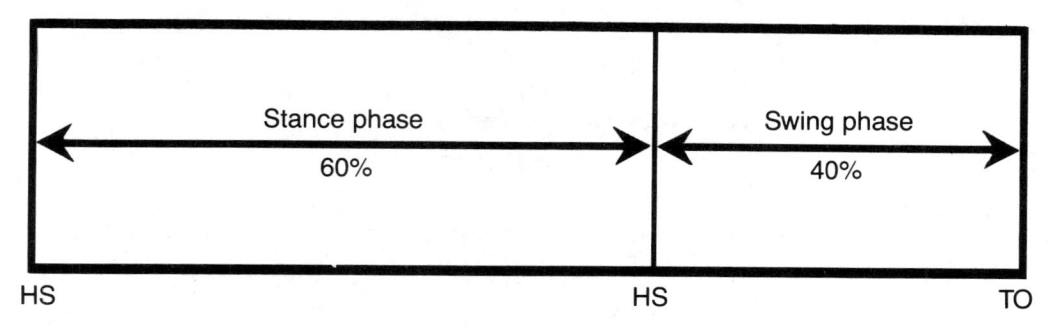

Figure 11.3. The complete gait cycle.

11-15
This chapter concerns the effect of rearfoot pathology on the gait cycle. In order to appreciate pathologic effects, it is necessary to review and learn well the normal joint motion which should occur during the gait cycle.

toe off, same,
heel strike, same

Since we will examine the effect of rearfoot pathology in the gait cycle, the joint motion on which we will concentrate is that of the STJ.

11-16
During the first half of the swing phase, the STJ (*pronates/supinates*).

11-17
This pronation allows the foot to clear the ground by effectively shortening the limb length.

pronates

11-18
During the last half of the swing phase of gait, the STJ (*pronates/supinates*).

11-19
This supination *stabilizes* the foot in preparation for heel strike.

supinates

11-20
So, during the first half of the swing phase, the STJ is _____ing.

During the last half of the swing phase, the STJ is _____ing (Fig. 11.4).

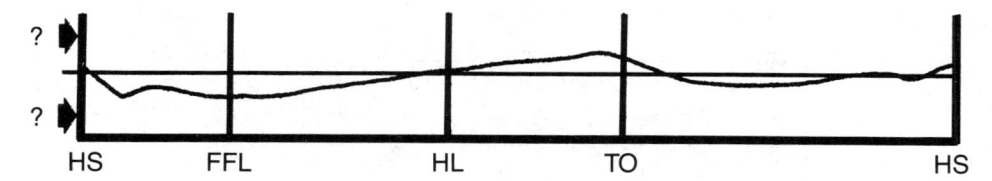

Figure 11.4. STJ motion during the gait cycle.

pronat(ing), supinat(ing)	**11-21** Swing phase supination occurs in order to _____ the foot for heel strike. Swing phase pronation occurs in order to effectively (*lengthen/ shorten*) the lower limb.
stabilize, shorten	**11-22** At heel strike, the STJ is in a slightly supinated position. Between heel strike and the opposite foot's toe off, i.e., the _____ period, the STJ is (*supinating/pronating*) in order to make the foot a (*rigid lever/mobile adaptor*).
contact, pronating, mobile adaptor	**11-23** During the contact period, the STJ pronation makes the foot a better mobile adaptor because STJ pronation makes the foot more flexible.
	11-24 In contrast to the contact period, during the midstance and propulsive periods, the STJ is (*pronating/supinating*).
supinating	**11-25** As opposed to the contact period, during the midstance and propulsive periods, STJ motion makes the foot a more (*rigid lever/mobile adaptor*).
rigid lever	**11-26** So, during the contact period, the STJ (*pronates/supinates*). During the midstance and propulsive periods, the STJ (*pronates/supinates*).
pronates, supinates	**11-27** Recall the following from Chapter 4. By having the foot function as a rigid lever during the time immediately preceding toe off, the weight of the body is propelled off of that limb with the greatest efficiency. If the STJ was, instead, pronating during propulsion and in a pronated position at toe off, the foot would become more of a mobile adaptor (i.e., a "loose bag of bones"). Therefore, it would take more muscle energy to propel the weight of the body off of such a platform. Some types of foot pathology cause abnormal pronation during propulsion and a pronated position at the end of propulsion. As a result, there is significant foot and leg fatigue secondary to overuse of muscles. Additionally, abnormal pronation during the propulsive period causes *hypermobility* and *abnormal shearing forces* to occur. (In case you're wondering, the reason that we are not extremely concerned about abnormal STJ pronation in the other periods of the stance phase of gait is that during those times, hypermobility and abnormal shear forces are relatively much less significant because weight is more evenly distributed across the whole foot.)

11-28

Recall that in Chapter 4, we defined *hypermobility* as *an unstable state of joints which are supposed to be stable.*

The result of hypermobility is joint subluxation.

This occurs because forces, which the normally stable joint is able to resist, are now capable of acting on and deforming an unstable (or _____) joint.

hypermobile

11-29

Abnormal pronation during the propulsive period causes hypermobility and abnormal _____ forces to occur.

shearing

11-30

The hypermobility causes joint _____.

subluxation

11-31

Recall that the abnormal shearing forces produced by abnormal propulsive pronation occur between the skin and bones of the forefoot, in particular, the metatarsal heads.

The frequent result of these abnormal irritative forces is the generation of hyperkeratotic callus tissue (Fig. 11.5). However, one may correctly extrapolate that other conditions produced by abnormal irritative forces between the skin and bones—e.g., *adventitious bursal formation, hemorrhage,* and *fibrosis*—may also occur.

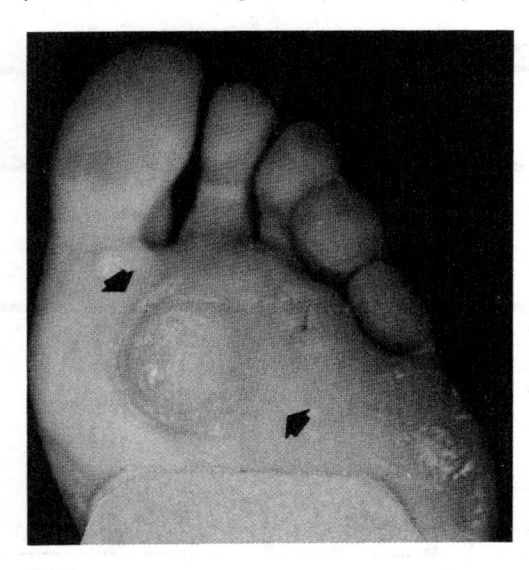

Figure 11.5.
Hyperkeratotic callus tissue.

11-32

Abnormal propulsive pronation produces abnormal shearing forces between the skin and bones of the _____.

11-33

The bones, in particular, which are involved are the _____ _____.

forefoot

metatarsal heads

hyperkeratotic or callus

11-34
The frequently seen result of this type of abnormal shearing force is the generation of _____ tissue.

11-35
Additionally, abnormal shearing forces in the propulsive period may cause the development of hemorrhage, fibrosis, or adventitious bursa.

11-36
Now that the consequences of abnormal STJ pronation during the propulsive period have been examined, we can isolate the major causes of abnormal propulsive STJ pronation.

11-37
In patients with rearfoot varus, the STJ remains in a pronated position from heel strike until the end of the midstance period (Fig. 11.6). Then, during the propulsive period, the STJ supinates. This supination, however, is not enough to bring the STJ from a pronated to a neutral or supinated position.

Read the above again, and visualize the STJ's motion and position during the stance phase of gait. Think about this situation juxtaposed with the normal STJ motion expected.

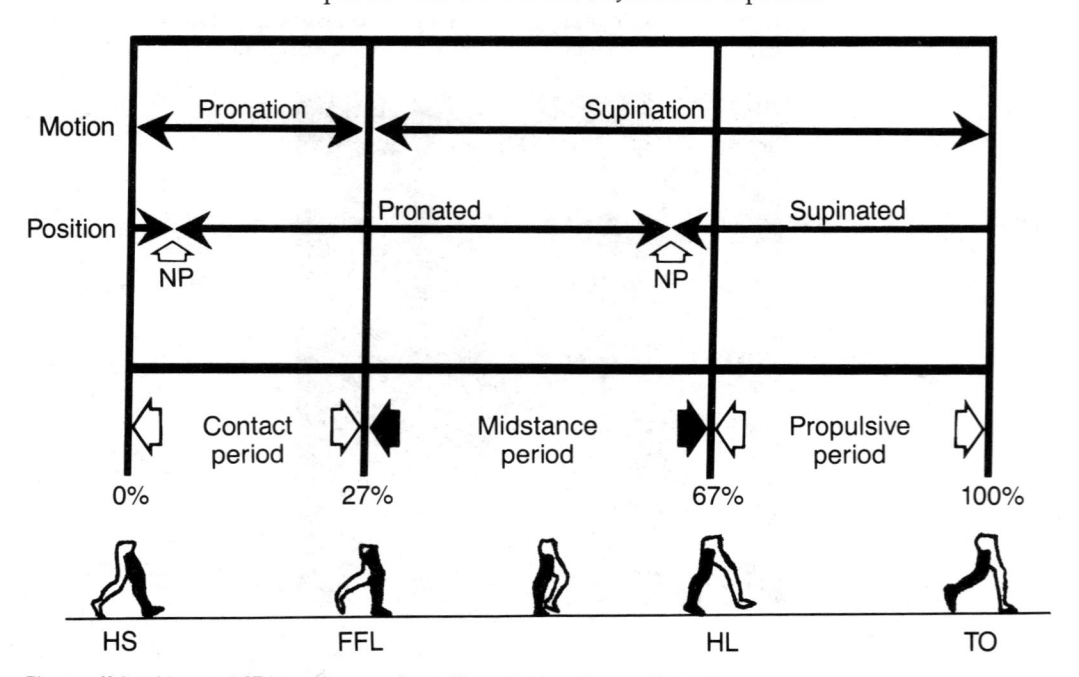

Figure 11.6. Normal STJ motion and position during the gait cycle.

11-38
In the normal foot, the STJ pronates throughout the contact period and then supinates throughout the _____ and _____ periods.

11-39
In a patient with rearfoot varus, the STJ _____ throughout the contact period and _____ throughout the midstance period.

midstance, propulsive

11-40
Then, during the propulsive period, the rearfoot varus patient's STJ will _____.

pronates, pronates

11-41
Is this supination enough to take the STJ to a neutral or a supinated position?

supinate

11-42
Because the rearfoot varus patient has abnormal STJ pronation occurring during propulsion, one could expect there to be _____ and abnormal _____ forces within the forefoot.

no

11-43
In the patient with an equinus-type foot (inadequate ankle joint dorsiflexion with the knee extended), STJ pronation during the propulsive period is also observed (as long as the heel contacts the ground at the beginning of the contact period).

hypermobility, shearing

This occurs (basically) so that the foot will become more mobile and allow the forefoot to stay in contact with and accommodate to the supporting surface for a longer time.

While this type of compensation causes some STJ pronation during the contact and midstance phases, there is massive STJ pronation that occurs just before propulsion begins.

Because of this, the tendency for STJ subluxation at the beginning of the propulsive period is great in the patient with an equinus-type foot.

The STJ remains in a pronated position during propulsion.

11-44
So, the two types of rearfoot pathology which cause STJ pronation during the propulsive periods are _____ _____ and the _____-type of foot.

rearfoot varus, equinus

11-45
(Fig. 11.7) In both conditions, during the contact and midstance periods, the STJ _____.

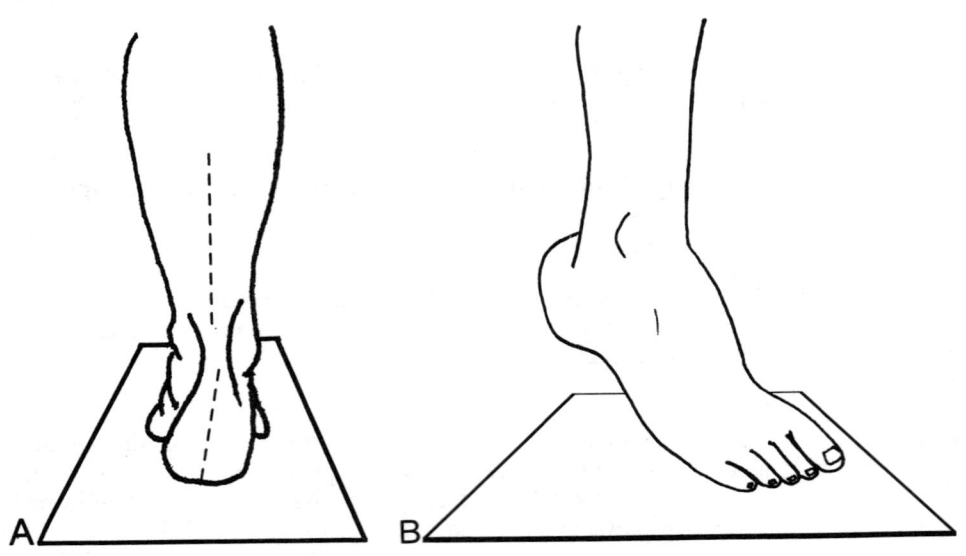

Figure 11.7. A, Rearfoot varus. B, Talipes equinus.

pronates

11-46
Just before the propulsive period, the equinus-type foot will undergo massive _____ _____.

This leads to a great tendency for STJ _____ to occur at the beginning of the propulsive period.

STJ pronation, subluxation

11-47
In the rearfoot varus patient, during the propulsive period, the STJ will _____.

supinate

11-48
In both the rearfoot varus and equinus patients, the STJ will remain in a _____ position during the propulsive period.

pronated

11-49
In rearfoot valgus and tarsal coalitions, there is *persistent STJ pronation* throughout the entire stance phase of gait.

11-50
Recall that rearfoot valgus of over 2° and less than 10° will cause the STJ to pronate maximally.

If the rearfoot valgus measures 10° or over, then the STJ will pronate 0° to 3° from its neutral position.

Tarsal coalitions cause pronation throughout the entire gait cycle to decrease STJ _____.

11: EFFECTS OF REARFOOT PATHOLOGY ON THE GAIT CYCLE

11-51
So, there are four main types of rearfoot pathology which will cause the STJ to be in a pronated position during the propulsive period. These are: rearfoot _____, rearfoot _____, tarsal _____, and an _____-type foot.

irritation

11-52
The condition which causes massive STJ pronation just prior to the propulsive period is _____.

varus, valgus, coalitions, equinus

11-53
The condition in which there is some STJ supination during the propulsive period (although the STJ still remains in a pronated position) is _____ _____.

equinus

11-54
The conditions which cause STJ pronation throughout the entire stance phase are _____ _____ and _____ _____.

rearfoot varus

11-55
Recall that for an equinus foot to maintain the STJ in a pronated position during propulsion, it is necessary for the heel to contact the ground at the beginning of the contact period.

tarsal coalition, rearfoot valgus

If the equinus is so severe that the heel does not contact the ground at the beginning of the contact period, the ground force does not resist the STJ supinator muscles.

This results in a supinated deformity of the foot.

11-56
The only rearfoot pathology which we have discussed, which is capable of causing a supinated deformity of the foot, is in an _____-type foot in which the heel (*does/does not*) touch the ground at the beginning of the contact period.

11-57
All rearfoot pathology which causes the STJ to be pronated during the propulsive period will cause _____, especially in the forefoot, as well as abnormal _____ forces which are also concentrated about the forefoot.

equinus, does not

11-58
This concludes this chapter.

hypermobility, shearing

In Chapter 16, the effect of forefoot pathology on the gait cycle will be examined. At that time, you may want to review this chapter as there are some interesting similarities.

Questions

FRAMES 11-19 AND 11-21

1. Swing phase supination occurs in order to effectively *shorten* the lower limb.
   a. true
   b. false

FRAME 11-22

2. At heel strike, the STJ is in a:
   a. slightly pronated position
   b. slightly supinated position
   c. neutral position
   d. either a or b
   e. either b or c

FRAME 11-25

3. The STJ normally supinates during the:
   a. contact period
   b. midstance period
   c. propulsive period
   d. a and b
   e. b and c

FRAME 11-27

4. Hypermobility and shearing forces secondary to abnormal STJ pronation are most significant during the:
   a. contact period
   b. midstance period
   c. propulsive period
   d. stance phase
   e. swing phase

FRAME 11-28

5. Hypermobility results in:
   a. STJ pronation
   b. abnormal shearing forces
   c. joint subluxation
   d. a and b
   e. b and c

FRAME 11-31

6. Abnormal shearing forces can produce:
   a. adventitious bursa
   b. fibrosis
   c. hemorrhage
   d. a and b
   e. a, b, and c

11: EFFECTS OF REARFOOT PATHOLOGY ON THE GAIT CYCLE

FRAME 11-37

7. The STJ pronates throughout the contact and midstance periods and supinates some during the propulsive period in patients that have:
   a. rearfoot varus
   b. rearfoot valgus
   c. tarsal coalition
   d. a and b
   e. b and c

FRAME 11-43

8. Massive STJ pronation during the propulsive period is observed in a patient with:
   a. rearfoot valgus
   b. rearfoot varus
   c. tibial varum
   d. tarsal coalition
   e. equinus-type foot

FRAME 11-49

9. *Persistent STJ pronation* throughout the stance phase of gait occurs with:
   a. rearfoot varus
   b. rearfoot valgus
   c. tarsal coalition
   d. a and b
   e. b and c

FRAME 11-55

10. A severe equinus deformity, which does not allow the heel to touch the ground at the beginning of the contact period, will:
    a. cause a pronated deformity of the foot
    b. cause a supinated deformity of the foot
    c. not have any effect on the position of the foot
    d. cause a compensatory plantarflexed first ray
    e. cause a compensatory forefoot valgus

Answers

1. b	4. c	7. a	10. b
2. b	5. e	8. e	
3. e	6. e	9. e	

CHAPTER 12

Normal Midtarsal Joint Function and Measurement

- MTJ review
- STJ position's effect on MTJ range of motion
- clinical index of MTJ position—definition and measurement
- abnormal MTJ motion—effects in the gait cycle

12-1
Before we discuss function, let's briefly review the MTJ. The MTJ has (*one/two/three*) separate axes.

12-2

two

The two axes of the MTJ are the longitudinal axis and the _____ axis (Fig. 12.1).

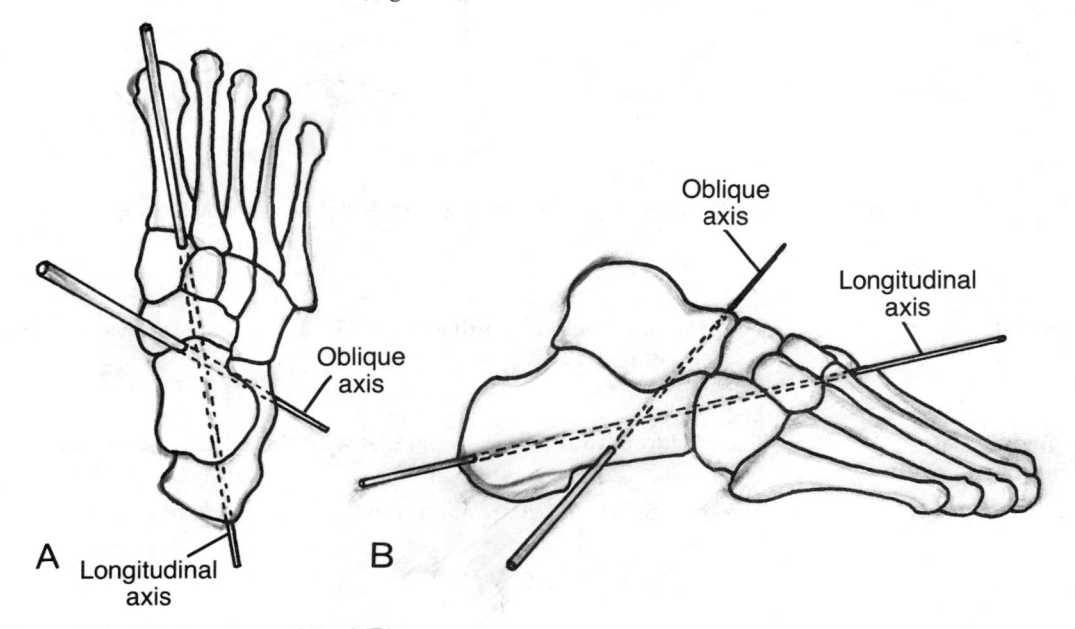

Figure 12.1. The two axes of the MTJ.

oblique

12-3
Although, in reality, triplane motion occurs about both MTJ axes, some planes of motion are so small as to be clinically insignificant.

Triplane motion about the axes of the MTJ is important in purely academic circles, however, *for practical purposes,* we will talk about only one or two planes of motion about a particular MTJ axis.

12-4
(Fig. 12.2) Recall that the *longitudinal axis* is (just about) parallel with both the transverse and sagittal planes.

Because of this spatial orientation, we know that (for practical purposes) motion about the longitudinal axis of the MTJ will only occur in the _____ plane.

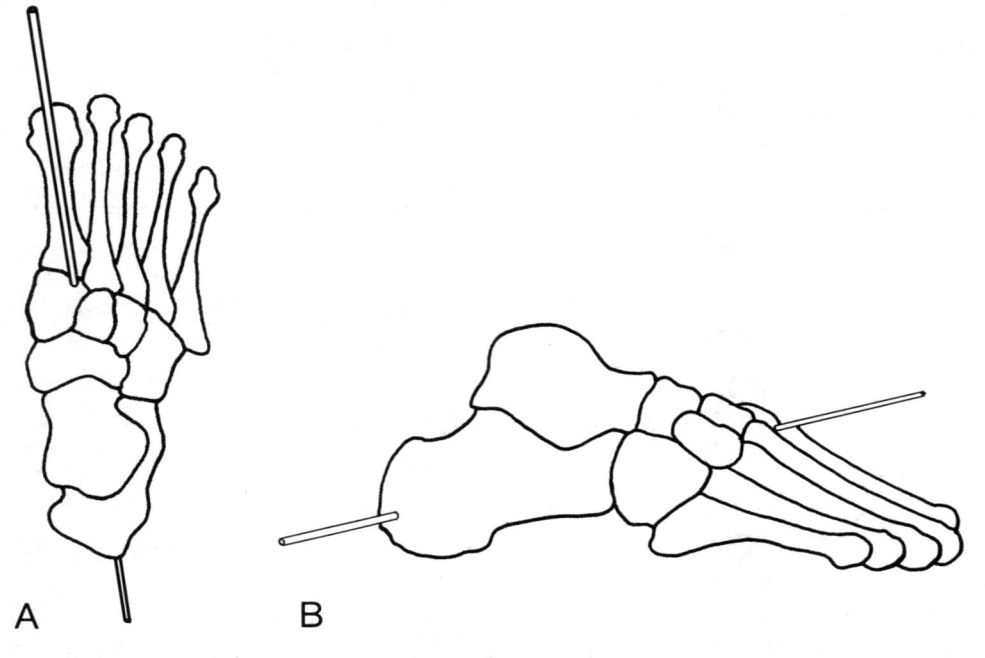

Figure 12.2. *A,* A dorsal view of the MTJ longitudinal axis. *B,* A lateral view of the MTJ longitudinal axis.

frontal

12-5
The frontal plane motion that the MTJ _____ axis allows is called _____ and _____.

longitudinal, inversion, eversion

12-6
The MTJ longitudinal axis is parallel with the _____ and _____ planes.

The motion which occurs about it is _____ plane motion.

12: NORMAL MIDTARSAL JOINT FUNCTION AND MEASUREMENT

transverse, sagittal, frontal

12-7
Since the MTJ longitudinal axis allows only frontal plane motion, it follows that the other MTJ axis, i.e., the _____ axis (Fig. 12.3), might allow both sagittal and transverse plane motion.

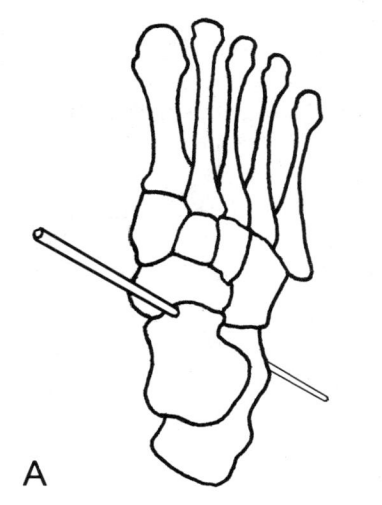

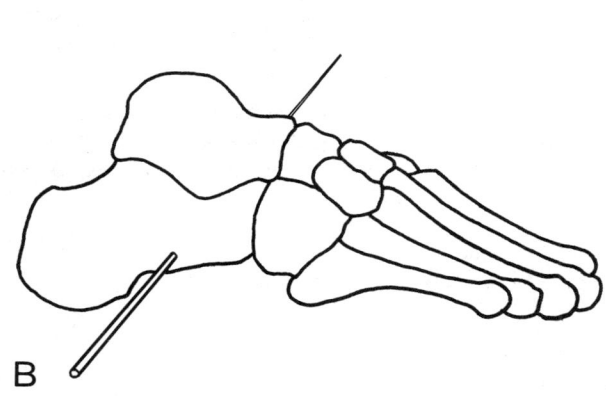

Figure 12.3 A.

Figure 12.3 B.

oblique

12-8
In fact, motion in three planes *can* occur with contributions from the two axes of the MTJ.

Sagittal plane motion occurs about the MTJ _____ axis.

Frontal plane motion occurs about the MTJ _____ axis.

Transverse plane motion occurs about the MTJ _____ axis.

oblique, longitudinal, oblique

12-9
It is important to be easily aware of the specific axis and its associated motion in order to understand MTJ function during the gait cycle.

12-10
Since two planes of motion occur about the MTJ oblique axis, it is necessary to know which motions are *coupled*.

An easy mnemonic to remember these coupled motions is "pad and dab."

With *p*lantarflexion, *ad*duction also occurs.

Simultaneously, with *d*orsiflexion, *ab*duction occurs.

12-11
Motion is coupled about the MTJ _____ axis.

Plantarflexion occurs with _____ and dorsiflexion occurs with _____.

oblique, adduction, abduction

12-12
The two motions which occur about the MTJ longitudinal axis are _____ and _____.

These are _____ plane motions.

inversion, eversion, frontal

12-13
Both sagittal and transverse plane motion occur about the MTJ oblique axis (Fig. 12.4) because of its spatial orientation; it is almost *parallel with the frontal plane* and almost *equally angulated from the sagittal and transverse planes* about 55°.

(Actually, the average angulation of the MTJ oblique axis is 57° from the sagittal plane and 52° from the transverse plane. For our purposes, however, it is easier and completely adequate to remember 55°.)

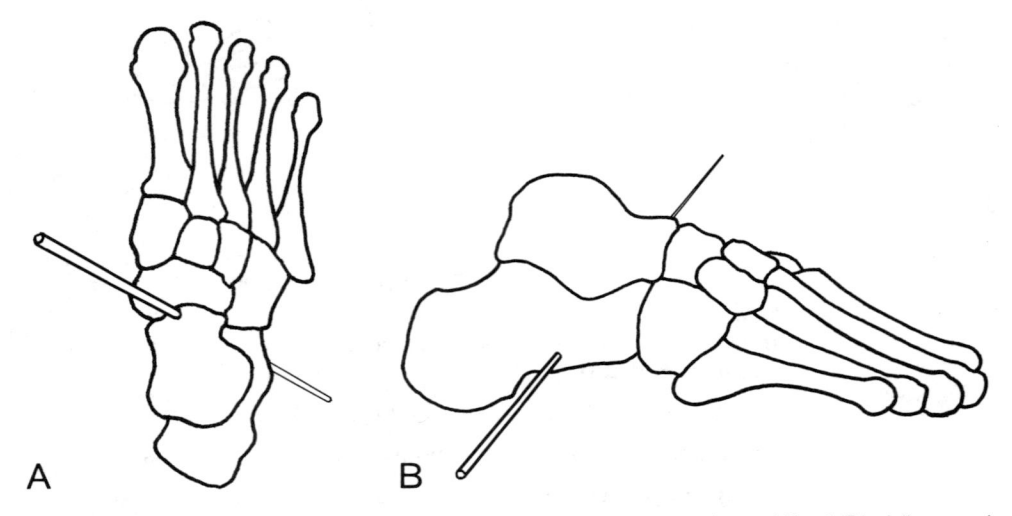

Figure 12.4 *A*, A dorsal view of the MTJ oblique axis. *B*, A lateral view of the MTJ oblique axis.

12-14
These relative angulations make sense since the only plane of motion *not* available at the MTJ oblique axis is the _____ plane.

Motion cannot occur in a plane if the joint axis is (*perpendicular/parallel*) to that plane.

frontal, parallel

12-15
While the ROM of the MTJ oblique axis is unknown, the MTJ's *longitudinal axis* has an average ROM of about 4° to 6°.

One thing that is very important to remember for clinical application is that *the MTJ's total ROM is dependent upon the STJ's position.*

12-16

The reason for this can be found by examining the shape and configuration of the two proximal articular facets that compose the MTJ.

The longitudinal axes of the articular facets are just about parallel when the STJ is maximally pronated. This allows a certain congruity to the two joints which compose the MTJ—the talonavicular and calcaneocuboid joints—similar to the axis of a hinge.

As the STJ goes from a maximally pronated position toward a more supinated position, the longitudinal axes of the two joints progressively diverge from one another (Fig. 12.5). Congruity is progressively lost, and, along with it, ROM progressively decreases.

This is an important concept. Please reread this frame slowly and visualize in your mind the position of the articular facets as the STJ goes from a maximally pronated to a maximally supinated position.

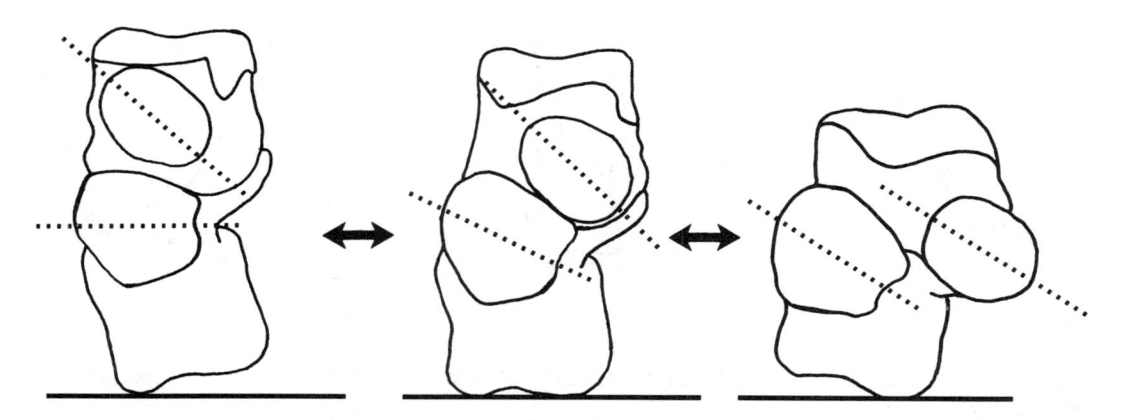

Figure 12.5. When the STJ is in its maximally pronated position (far right), the longitudinal axes of the articular facets are lined up close to parallel with one another. In the STJ neutral position, the angulation between the longitudinal axes has increased. Further divergence of the axes are noted on the far left where the STJ is in its maximally supinated position.

12-17

The MTJ oblique axis has motion available in two planes: the _____ and the _____ planes.

sagittal, transverse

12-18

The MTJ oblique axis is angulated _____° from both of these planes.

55

12-19

Motion about the MTJ oblique axis cannot occur in the _____ plane since the axis is (*perpendicular/parallel*) to that plane.

frontal, parallel

12-20

The average ROM for the MTJ oblique axis is unknown; however, the average ROM for the MTJ longitudinal axis is _____° to _____°.

4 (to) 6

12-21

Before further discussing the MTJ, it should be pointed out that *the standard clinical index for MTJ position is the relationship of the plantar plane of the five metatarsal heads to the plantar plane of the rearfoot when the MTJ is maximally pronated about both of its axes* (Fig. 12.6).

The plantar plane of the five metatarsal heads is the same as the plantar plane of the forefoot.

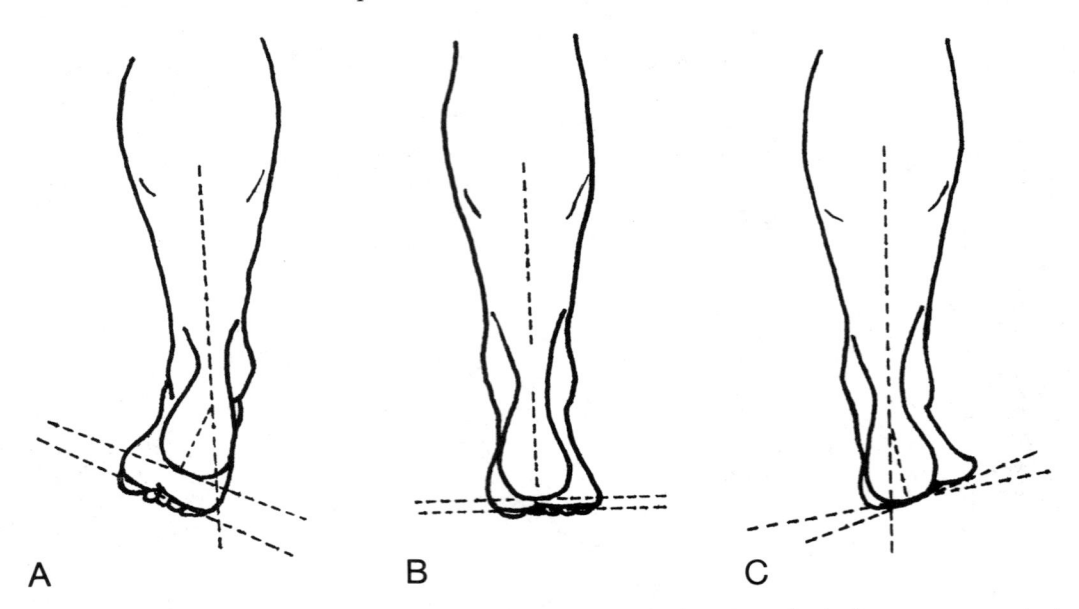

Figure 12.6. Observation of the plantar planes of the forefoot and rearfoot allows assessment of MTJ position.

12-22

The standard clinical index for MTJ position is the relationship between the _____ plane of the five metatarsal heads (i.e., the _____ plane of the _____) and the plantar plane of the _____.

The plantar plane of the rearfoot is usually derived as a perpendicular to the posterior calcaneal bisection. *The relation between the plantar plane of the forefoot with the plantar plane of the rearfoot helps us assess the MTJ position clinically.*

plantar, plantar, forefoot, rearfoot

12-23

The plantar plane of the rearfoot is usually derived as a perpendicular to the posterior calcaneal bisection. The relationship between the plantar plane of the forefoot with the plantar plane of the rearfoot helps us to assess the MTJ position clinically.

12-24

When we say that the MTJ is *"locked"* or *"loaded,"* we are referring to a MTJ in which both axes are maximally pronated.

12: NORMAL MIDTARSAL JOINT FUNCTION AND MEASUREMENT 141

12-25
A locked MTJ, i.e., an MTJ in which the longitudinal and oblique axes are fully _____, is the standard by which the MTJ position is evaluated clinically.

Recall that we said the total MTJ ROM is determined by the position of the _____ joint.

pronated, subtalar

12-26
The foot is most flexible (i.e., the best mobile adaptor) when the STJ is maximally _____.

pronated

12-27
Therefore, it is not surprising that the MTJ has its *greatest* ROM when the STJ is _____ _____.

maximally pronated

12-28
Conversely, the foot is least flexible (i.e., most rigid) when the STJ is maximally _____.

This would then correspond to the time when the MTJ has its (*greatest/average/smallest*) ROM.

supinated, smallest

12-29
To correlate these relative MTJ ROMs with what is observed clinically, it is first necessary to appreciate the fact that in the normal foot, *when the STJ is in its neutral position and the MTJ is maximally pronated (i.e., "_____" or "_____"), the plantar plane of the forefoot is parallel with the plantar plane of the rearfoot.*

loaded, locked

12-30
That is to say that in the normal foot, when the MTJ axes are fully pronated, the plantar planes of the forefoot and rearfoot are parallel with each other only when the STJ is in its _____ position.

neutral

12-31
(Fig. 12.7) When the STJ is maximally supinated and the MTJ's ROM is (*increased/unchanged/decreased*), the plantar plane of the forefoot is inverted relative to the plantar plane of the rearfoot when the MTJ is maximally _____.

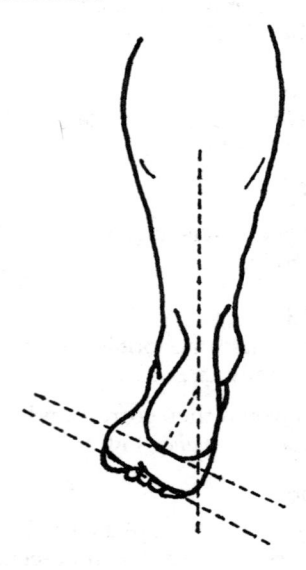

Figure 12.7.

decreased, pronated

12-32
The decreased MTJ ROM that occurs with STJ _____ does not allow the plantar plane of the forefoot to evert enough so that it becomes parallel with the plantar plane of the _____ when the MTJ is loaded.

supination, rearfoot

12-33
(Fig. 12.8) When the STJ is maximally pronated, the MTJ's ROM is (*increased/the same/decreased*) and the (plantar plane of the) forefoot becomes everted relative to the (plantar plane of the) rearfoot.

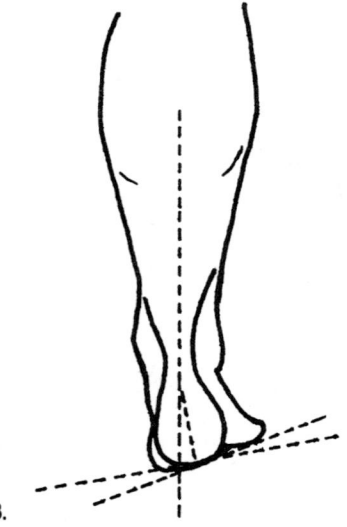

Figure 12.8.

12-34

The MTJ ROM (and its relationship with STJ position) is very important clinically.

The MTJ that functions normally allows the forefoot to become a mobile adaptor when necessary during the contact period and, likewise, a progressively more and more rigid lever during the midstance and propulsive periods of gait.

If the MTJ has a larger relative ROM than it should during the midstance or propulsive periods, the muscles controlling the forefoot position will have to overwork in an attempt to stabilize the forefoot. The muscles' force vectors may also change, thus causing powerful *deforming forces* on many foot joints.

The force vectors which can occur with abnormal MTJ function can cause *subluxation* and/or *dislocation* of the affected joints. Because these muscles must overwork in these situations, *foot and leg fatigue* are not unusual findings in cases of forefoot pathology.

increased

12-35
So, in a patient with rearfoot varus, where the STJ is in an abnormally pronated position during the stance phase of gait, one would expect the MTJ ROM to be (*increased/the same/decreased*).

increased

12-36
In the rearfoot varus patient, one would expect to see foot and leg fatigue because of the abnormal STJ pronation as well as the abnormally (*increased/decreased*) MTJ ROM.

increased

12-37
In a patient with any condition which causes abnormal STJ pronation throughout the stance period, one could expect foot and/or leg _____ and possibly joint _____ and/or _____.

fatigue, subluxation, dislocation

12-38
This is exemplary of the extreme significance of MTJ function and its integral relationship with STJ position (and, therefore, function.) These interrelationships will be further explored in Chapter 14, and clinical problems will be presented to help integrate the material.

12-39
Recall that to assess the MTJ position, we evaluate the relationship of the _____ plane of the _____ relative to the _____ plane of the _____ with the MTJ in its maximally _____ position and the STJ in its neutral position.

**plantar, forefoot,
plantar, rearfoot,
pronated**

12-40

(Fig. 12.9) In the normal foot, these relationships are as follows.

With the STJ neutral, the plantar plane of the forefoot is _____ relative to the plantar plane of the rearfoot.

When the STJ is maximally supinated, the MTJ's ROM is (*increased/the same/decreased*) and the plantar plane of the forefoot is _____ relative to the plantar plane of the rearfoot.

Finally, when the STJ is maximally pronated, the MTJ causes the plantar plane of the forefoot to be _____ relative to the plantar plane of the rearfoot and the MTJ's total ROM to be (*increased/the same/decreased*).

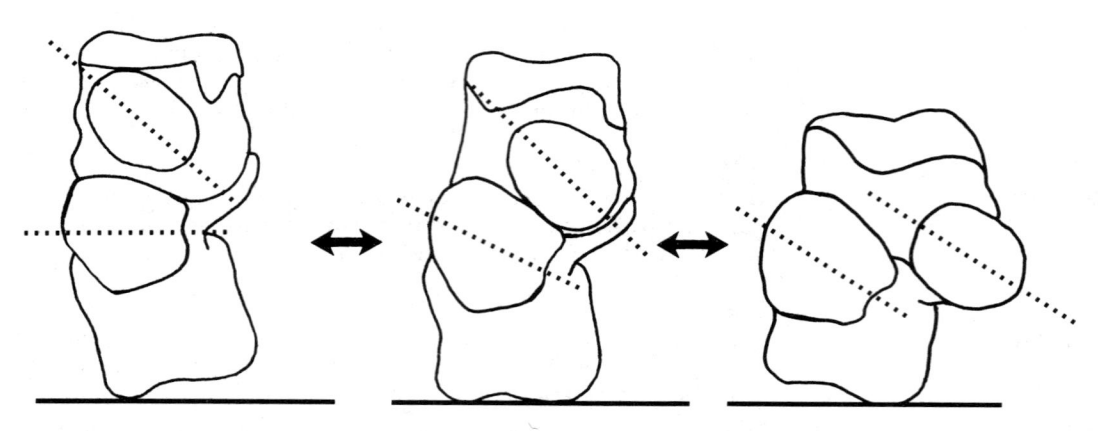

Figure 12.9. The STJ position influences the MTJ ROM, and, therefore, the relationship between the plantar planes of the forefoot and rearfoot (with the MTJ maximally pronated about both its axes).

**parallel, decreased,
inverted, everted,
increased**

12-41

There are two methods commonly employed to measure the forefoot to rearfoot relationship (i.e., the MTJ).

Both utilize the posterior calcaneal bisection as a reference point, since the plantar plane of the rearfoot is (*parallel/perpendicular*) to the calcaneal bisection.

perpendicular

12-42

One method of measuring the MTJ utilizes an instrument called variably a *goniometer* or *tractograph*.

When using this instrument, the STJ is placed in its neutral position and the MTJ is loaded (i.e., maximally _____). While the foot is maintained in this position, the instrument is placed in the frontal plane across the forefoot. One arm of the instrument is positioned perpendicular to the posterior calcaneal bisection while the other arm is held against the first and fifth metatarsal heads.

The goniometer is then removed, and the angle is read. This angle reflects the relationship of the plantar plane of the forefoot to the plantar plane of the rearfoot.

12: NORMAL MIDTARSAL JOINT FUNCTION AND MEASUREMENT

pronated

12-43
A two-armed instrument used for measuring the relationship of the forefoot to the rearfoot is called a _____ or _____.

goniometer, tractograph

12-44
This instrument is used to measure the relationship of the forefoot to the rearfoot, thus giving an index of the position of the _____ joint.

midtarsal

12-45
The other instrument that is used for measuring the relative position of the forefoot to the rearfoot is called, appropriately, a *forefoot measuring device*.

12-46
So, the two instruments that can be used for measuring the MTJ position are the _____ and the _____ _____ _____.

goniometer or tractograph, forefoot measuring device

12-47
The forefoot measuring device also requires the STJ to be held in its neutral position while the MTJ is maximally pronated.

The open slit is then positioned over the calcaneal bisection and the flat side of the protractor is placed so that it lines up along the plantar plane of the forefoot.

The angulation between forefoot and rearfoot is then read on the protractor scale.

(The author prefers using the goniometer for this measurement as the forefoot measuring device is, for some people, difficult to use and offers no advantage over the goniometric method.)

12-48
The average MTJ longitudinal axis ROM is _____° to _____° of motion in the _____ plane.

4, 6, frontal

12-49
By using this type of instrumentation, one can readily observe that with pronation of the STJ, the MTJ longitudinal axis ROM (*increases/stays the same/decreases*), and the forefoot becomes relatively (*inverted/parallel/everted*) relative to the rearfoot.

increases, everted

12-50
Likewise, one would expect that with the STJ maximally supinated, the forefoot would be relatively (*inverted/parallel/everted*) to the rearfoot with the total MTJ longitudinal axis ROM (*increasing/staying the same/decreasing*).

inverted, decreasing

12-51
Since position about the MTJ oblique axis cannot specifically be measured, one must rely on gross morphologic observations to assess its function.

One observation that is particularly useful is based on the fact that with STJ pronation, the coupled motions about the MTJ oblique axis (of dorsiflexion and _____) are increased.

abduction

12-52
Because of this, the forefoot can be seen to be relatively abducted on the rearfoot during weightbearing.

This is another sign that there is increased motion at the MTJ. It is, however, somewhat more subjective than the measurement of forefoot to rearfoot relationships and may not always be apparent even in extremely pronated feet.

12-53
This concludes the chapter. The following two chapters will examine normal and abnormal MTJ function in the gait cycle and in static stance.

Questions

FRAME 12-4

1. The longitudinal axis of the MTJ is just about parallel with the:
   a. sagittal plane
   b. transverse plane
   c. frontal plane
   d. a and b
   e. b and c

FRAMES 12-4 AND 12-5

2. Clinically, the MTJ longitudinal axis has about 4° to 6° of motion which is most apparent in the:
   a. sagittal plane
   b. frontal plane
   c. transverse plane
   d. a and b occur about equally
   e. a and c occur about equally

FRAME 12-10

3. In discussing the MTJ oblique axis, it is accurate to say that when *plantarflexion* occurs, so must:
   a. eversion
   b. inversion
   c. abduction
   d. adduction
   e. plantarflexion occurs without any coupled motion

FRAME 12-15

4. MTJ ROM is independent of STJ position.
   a. true
   b. false

FRAME 12-25

5. When evaluating the MTJ, it is imperative that the joint be maximally pronated about both its axes.
   a. true
   b. false

12: NORMAL MIDTARSAL JOINT FUNCTION AND MEASUREMENT

FRAME 12-30

6. In the normal foot, with the MTJ maximally pronated about both of its axes and the STJ in its neutral position, the plantar plane of the forefoot is:
   a. inverted to the plantar plane of the rearfoot
   b. parallel with the plantar plane of the rearfoot
   c. everted to the plantar plane of the rearfoot
   d. variably related to the plantar plane of the rearfoot
   e. none of the above is correct for the normal foot

FRAMES 12-32 AND 12-33

7. In a patient with a maximally pronated STJ, the MTJ ROM is _____, and the plantar plane of the forefoot becomes _____ relative to the plantar plane of the rearfoot.
   a. decreased, everted
   b. decreased, inverted
   c. increased, inverted
   d. increased, everted
   e. increased, parallel

FRAME 12-34

8. Increased MTJ ROM secondary to excessive STJ pronation during the midstance and propulsive periods may cause:
   a. greater flexibility in the foot
   b. foot and leg fatigue
   c. altered muscle force vectors creating deforming forces on many foot joints
   d. a and b
   e. a, b, and c

FRAMES 12-35 AND 12-36

9. In a rearfoot varus patient, during the stance phase, one would expect the MTJ ROM to be decreased.
   a. true
   b. false

FRAME 12-52

10. Increased motion at the MTJ can be observed indirectly by seeing the forefoot to be relatively adducted on the rearfoot.
    a. true
    b. false

Answers

1. d
2. b
3. d
4. b
5. a
6. b
7. d
8. e
9. b
10. b

CHAPTER
13

Normal Midtarsal Joint Function in the Gait Cycle

- review of effects of STJ position on MTJ function
- effect of ground reactive forces on the MTJ
- effect of muscular activity on the MTJ
- function of the MTJ during the gait cycle

13-1
To appreciate normal MTJ function in the gait cycle, it is necessary to remember how integrally related MTJ ROM (and, therefore, function) is to _____ position.

STJ

13-2

Before we begin to discuss the normal MTJ function during the gait cycle, let's review the effects of the STJ position on MTJ motion during gait (Fig 13.1).

Recall that at the beginning of the contact period, the STJ is slightly (*pronated/supinated*).

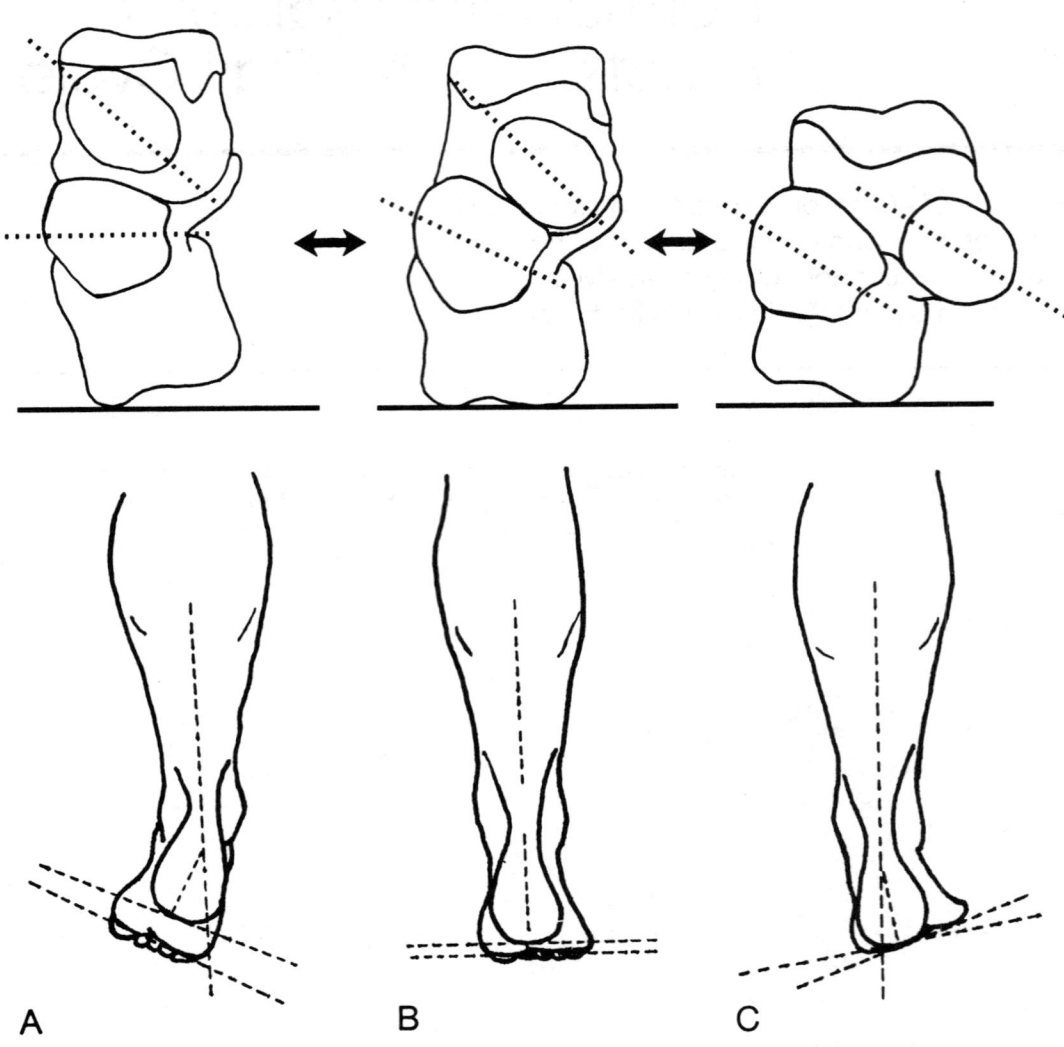

Figure 13.1. (All illustrations of the foot reflect the MTJ maximally pronated about both of its axes.) When the STJ is in a supinated position, as in A, the MTJ's ROM is maximally reduced. As the STJ progresses toward a pronated position, the MTJ ROM increases. As this occurs, the MTJ is able to pronate (evert) about its longitudinal axis more and more, thus moving the forefoot from an inverted position relative to the rearfoot when the STJ is maximally supinated to an everted position relative to the rearfoot when the STJ is maximally pronated. Note that when the STJ is in its neutral position, the plantar plane of the forefoot parallels that of the rearfoot.

supinated

13-3

Immediately after heel strike, the STJ reaches its neutral position as it (*supinates/pronates*).

13: NORMAL MIDTARSAL JOINT FUNCTION IN THE GAIT CYCLE

pronates

13-4
The reason that this pronation continues throughout the contact period (Fig. 13.2) is so the foot will become a more (*rigid lever/mobile adaptor*).

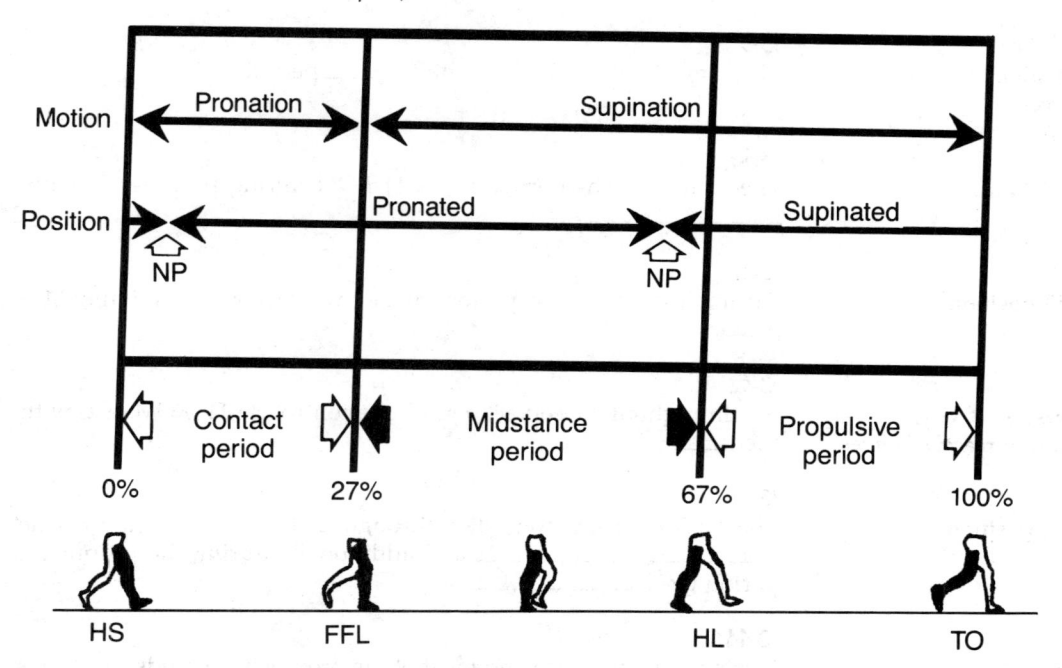

Figure 13.2. STJ motion during the gait cycle.

mobile adaptor

13-5
As the STJ pronates, the MTJ ROM (*increases/stays the same/decreases*).

increases

13-6
In fact, this increased MTJ ROM acts along with STJ _____ to make the foot a more mobile adaptor.

pronation

13-7
It is important to distinguish the different forces which act on the MTJ during the stance phase of gait.

Throughout the stance period, the MTJ *ROM* is passively controlled by the position of the STJ.

However, the MTJ *position* is controlled by ground reaction forces during the stance phase of gait and, additionally, by muscle activity during the propulsive period (Fig. 13.3).

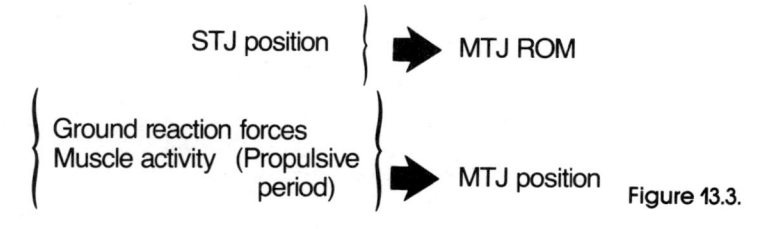

STJ position → MTJ ROM

Ground reaction forces
Muscle activity (Propulsive period) → MTJ position

Figure 13.3.

13-8
So, during the contact period, for example, one could say that the MTJ ROM is determined by the STJ _____ and that the MJT position is controlled by ground _____ _____.

position, reaction forces

13-9
The same would be true for the _____ period.

midstance

13-10
The factor which controls the MTJ *ROM* during propulsion is the _____ _____.

STJ position

13-11
During the *propulsive* period, what two factors control the MTJ *position*?

muscle activity, ground reaction forces

13-12
So, throughout the contact period, the control of MTJ *ROM* rests with the _____ _____.

STJ position

13-13
The MJT *position* is controlled throughout the stance period by the _____ _____ _____ and additionally during the propulsive period by _____ _____.

ground reaction forces, muscle activity

13-14
During the midstance and most of the propulsive periods, the STJ is (*supinating/pronating*).

This causes the available MTJ ROM to progressively (*increase/decrease*).

supinating, decrease

13-15
As these events occur, the foot becomes a more (*mobile adaptor/rigid lever*).

13: NORMAL MIDTARSAL JOINT FUNCTION IN THE GAIT CYCLE

rigid lever

13-16
Now that the gross function of the MTJ during the gait cycle has been examined, let's take a more detailed look at the individual MTJ axes during the gait cycle.

It is important to realize that while the MTJ has two separate axes (Fig. 13.4), these axes may not be doing the same thing at the same time. That is to say that one axis may be pronating at the same time the other is supinating.

(In the following discussion, we will use the terms pronating and supinating for both MTJ axes, as is done clinically. Realize that pronation for the MTJ longitudinal axis [*l.a.*] means eversion in practical terms. Likewise, for practical purposes, supination of the MTJ oblique axis [*o.a.*] means plantarflexion and adduction.)

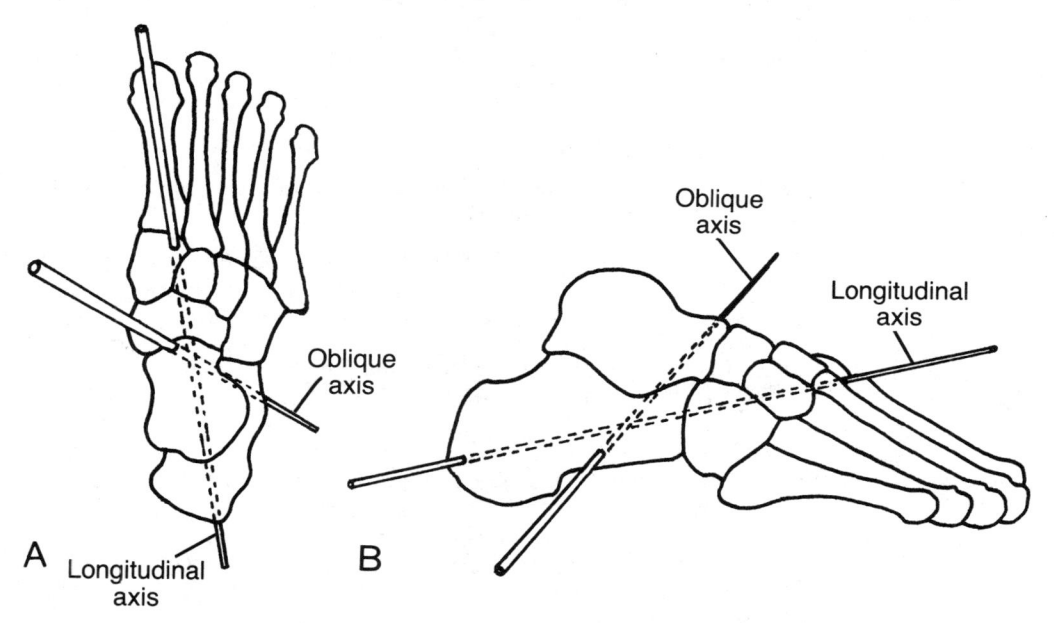

Figure 13.4. A, Dorsal view of the MTJ axes. B, Lateral view of the MTJ axes.

13-17
During the first half of the swing phase of gait, the STJ is (*pronating/supinating*).

pronating

13-18
This occurs in order to help the foot clear the ground.

Recall that the sagittal plane component of pronation is the motion of _____.

dorsiflexion

13-19
During the last half of the swing phase of gait, the STJ is (*pronating/supinating*).

supinating

13-20
(Fig. 13.5) This occurs to make the foot more rigid in preparation for heel strike.

As the foot is supinating, the muscles which dorsiflexed the foot during the first half of the swing phase are gradually relaxing—decelerating the foot as it goes through the sagittal plane component of supination (i.e., _____).

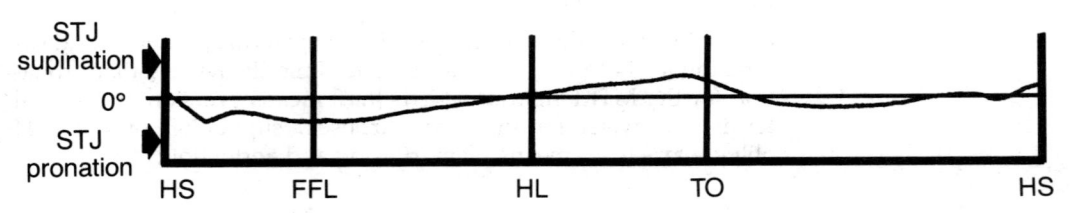

Figure 13.5. STJ motion and position during the stance phase of the gait cycle.

plantarflexion

13-21
The involved muscles also exert an effect on the MTJ's axes.

At heel strike, the *anterior tibial* muscle's pull is responsible for the supinated position of the MTJ l.a.

Thus, the forefoot is (*inverted/everted*) at heel strike.

inverted

13-22
At heel strike, while the MTJ l.a. is in a _____ position, the *peroneus tertius* and the *extensor digitorum longus* muscles maintain the MTJ o.a. in a pronated position.

supinated

13-23
All muscles mentioned above responsible for having pronated the MTJ o.a. (i.e., the _____ _____ and the _____ _____ _____) and having supinated the MTJ l.a. (i.e., the _____ _____) act together to decelerate the foot's plantarflexion.

peroneus tertius, extensor digitorum longus, anterior tibial

13-24
Without these muscles acting to _____ the plantarflexion of the foot, the foot would slap down onto the ground and encounter excessive shock which would then be transmitted up the lower extremity.

This is a point worth remembering as certain pathologic states (e.g., poliomyelitis, diabetic or alcoholic peripheral neuropathy) may allow this to occur.

decelerate

13-25
So then, to review, the muscles which cause the MTJ o.a. to be in a pronated position at heel strike are the _____ _____ _____ and the _____ _____.

extensor digitorum longus, peroneus tertius

13-26
The muscle which causes the MTJ l.a. to be in a supinated position at heel strike is the _____ _____.

13: NORMAL MIDTARSAL JOINT FUNCTION IN THE GAIT CYCLE

13-27
Pick from the following those adjectives which describe the forefoot relative to the rearfoot (based on MTJ position) at the time of heel strike:

anterior tibial

> dorsiflexed/plantarflexed
> inverted/everted
> abducted/adducted

13-28
Recall that the factor responsible for MTJ position during all of the stance phase is _____ _____ _____.

dorsiflexed, inverted, abducted

13-29
This is an important concept as it makes it much easier to understand what happens to the MTJ subsequent to heel strike.

ground reaction force

Once again, let's define the starting point at heel contact. Relative to the rearfoot, the forefoot is _____, _____, and _____.

13-30
That is to say, the MTJ o.a. is in a _____ position while the MTJ l.a. is in a _____ position.

dorsiflexed, abducted, inverted

13-31
Since the forefoot is inverted at heel strike, the lateral aspect of the forefoot comes into contact with the ground first.

pronated, supinated

The forefoot then absorbs the body's weight (through ground reactive force) progressively from lateral to medial. This is known as forefoot loading (Fig. 13.6).

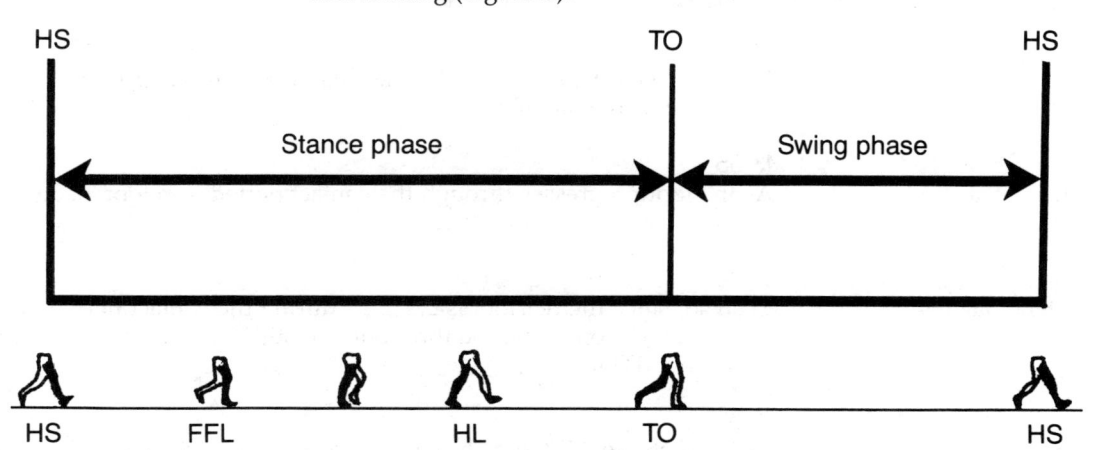

Figure 13.6. Forefoot loading (FFL) starts towards the end of the contact period.

13-32
While the forefoot absorbs the body's weight—i.e., _____ _____—from lateral to medial, the rearfoot is simultaneously in motion, pronating. In the process of rearfoot pronation, the clinical component most readily observed is eversion.

forefoot loading

13-33
The eversion of the rearfoot keeps the forefoot from pronating about the MTJ l.a.

Because of this, the forefoot ends up still supinated about the MTJ l.a. at the end of the contact period (Fig. 13.7).

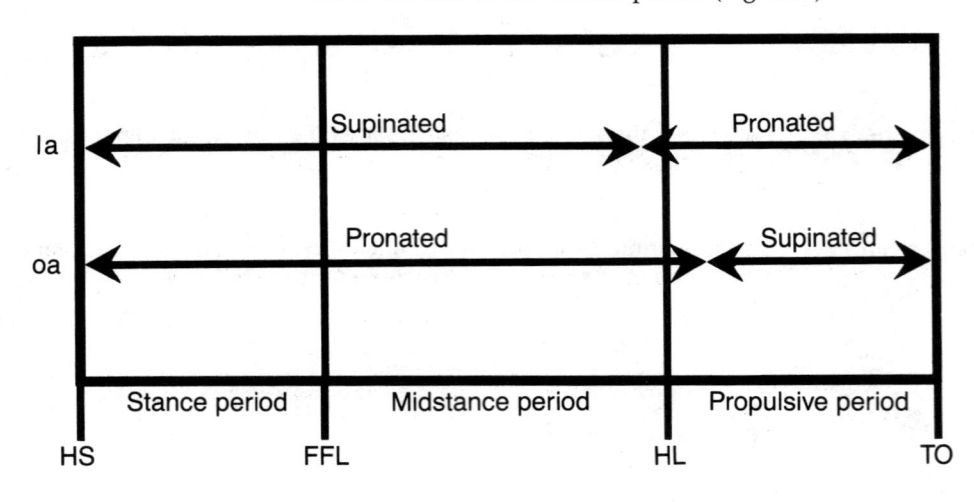

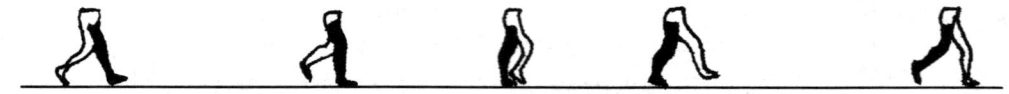

Figure 13.7. MTJ position about the longitudinal axis (l.a.) and the oblique axis (o.a.) during the stance phase of the gait cycle.

13-34
So, with regard to the MTJ l.a., at heel strike the forefoot is in a _____ position about it.

supinated

13-35
As the foot progresses through the contact period, forefoot loading occurs from _____ to _____.

lateral, medial

13-36
Even so, since the rearfoot is _____ during the contact period, at the end of the contact period the forefoot is still in a _____ position about the MTJ l.a.

everting (or pronating), supinated

13-37
Recall that the MTJ o.a. began the contact period in a _____ position.

pronated

13-38
Interestingly, the optimal position for the MTJ o.a. to assume in preparation for receiving weight is a _____ position.

pronated

13-39
Since forefoot loading starts during the contact period, the MTJ o.a. is maintained in a pronated position throughout the contact period of gait.

13: NORMAL MIDTARSAL JOINT FUNCTION IN THE GAIT CYCLE

13-40
Let's briefly review what happens to the STJ and MTJ during the contact period (Fig. 13.8).

At heel strike, the STJ is in a slightly _____ position.

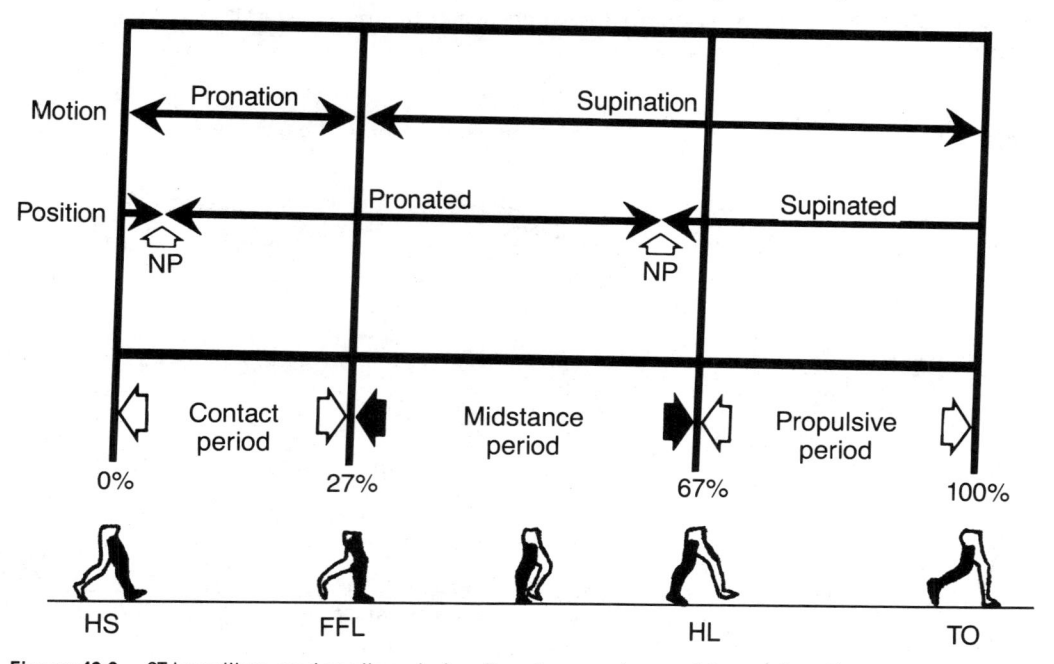

Figure 13.8. STJ position and motion during the stance phase of the gait cycle.

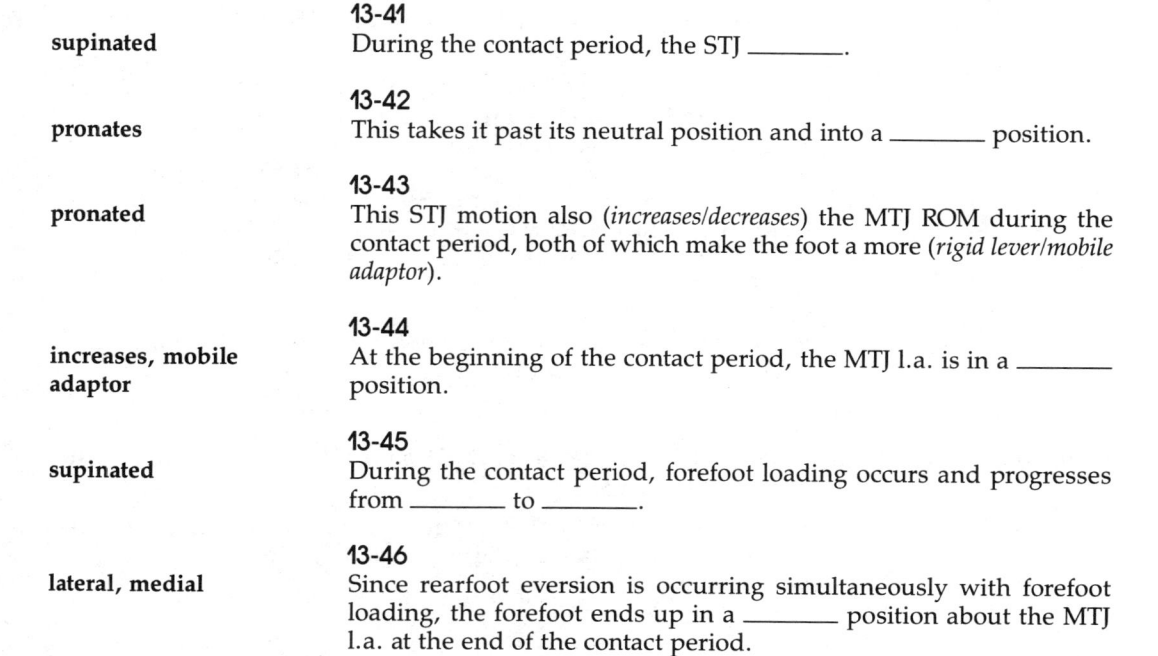

supinated

13-41
During the contact period, the STJ _____.

pronates

13-42
This takes it past its neutral position and into a _____ position.

pronated

13-43
This STJ motion also (*increases/decreases*) the MTJ ROM during the contact period, both of which make the foot a more (*rigid lever/mobile adaptor*).

increases, mobile adaptor

13-44
At the beginning of the contact period, the MTJ l.a. is in a _____ position.

supinated

13-45
During the contact period, forefoot loading occurs and progresses from _____ to _____.

lateral, medial

13-46
Since rearfoot eversion is occurring simultaneously with forefoot loading, the forefoot ends up in a _____ position about the MTJ l.a. at the end of the contact period.

13-47

supinated

The MTJ o.a. starts the contact period in a _____ position, which happens to be optimal for allowing the process of _____ _____.

13-48

pronated, forefoot loading

As the forefoot becomes weightbearing, the MTJ o.a. is maintained in a _____ position.

13-49

pronated

The MTJ o.a. ends the contact period of the stance phase in a _____ position.

13-50

pronated

Recall that the factor responsible for MTJ position during the midstance period is the _____ _____ _____.

13-51

ground reactive force

This force *maintains the MTJ o.a. in a pronated position throughout the midstance period.*

13-52

So, throughout both the contact and midstance periods, the MTJ o.a. remains in a _____ position.

13-53

pronated

Although the STJ pronates during the _____ period, it _____ during the midstance period and most of the propulsive period.

13-54

contact, supinates

During the midstance period, as the STJ supinates—thus inverting the foot—the forefoot, remaining in contact with the ground, is everted (i.e., pronated) about the MTJ l.a.

Keep in mind that the forefoot is not actually moving during this time. Its position is defined relative to the rearfoot. If the ground did not stabilize it, the forefoot would go along with the rearfoot and invert. However, since the forefoot *is* in contact with the ground, what actually happens is that the ground reactive force stops it from accompanying the rearfoot, and, thus, at the end of the midstance period, the forefoot ends up _____ about the MJT l.a.

13-55

pronated

So, at the end of the midstance period, the forefoot is in a _____ position about both the MTJ l.a. and MTJ o.a.

13-56

pronated

In fact, a pronated position about both MTJ axes is needed for the propulsive phase to begin.

Recall that the event that signals the end of the midstance period and the beginning of the propulsive period is the _____ _____ of the same foot.

13: NORMAL MIDTARSAL JOINT FUNCTION IN THE GAIT CYCLE

heel lift

13-57
If both axes of the MTJ were not fully pronated at this point (i.e., heel lift), the forefoot would not be stable enough to act as a rigid lever off of which the body could begin to propel.

13-58
To briefly review, the MTJ o.a. is in a _____ position during the contact period. At the end of the midstance period, the forefoot is in a _____ position about the MTJ o.a.

pronated, pronated

13-59
The MTJ l.a. is in a _____ position during the contact period and at the end of the midstance period is in a _____ position.

supinated, pronated

13-60
During the propulsive period, the body's weight must be transferred medially. Finally, the weight must be transferred over to the contra-lateral lower extremity.

The strong everters of the foot are the peroneal muscles. In order for them to work optimally in transferring body weight medially, the foot on which they exert their pull must be completely stabile.

Since the peroneals are everting the foot in order to transfer body weight _____, it follows that the foot must be maximally everted before these muscles can cause this effect.

medially

13-61
The peroneal muscles are strong _____ of the foot.

everters

13-62
If the forefoot was inverted, the peroneals would first have to maximally evert it before they could transfer the body weight _____.

This would be a suboptimal situation requiring a higher expenditure of energy to achieve the same goal.

medially

13-63
So, *throughout the propulsive period, the forefoot remains maximally pronated about the MTJ l.a.*

13-64
In the stance phase of gait, the MTJ l.a. starts out in a _____ position and ends up in a _____ position.

supinated, pronated

13-65
Recall that with STJ supination, there is also external rotation of the leg (Fig. 13.9).

Figure 13.9.
With CKC STJ supination, external rotation of the tibia (and leg) occurs.

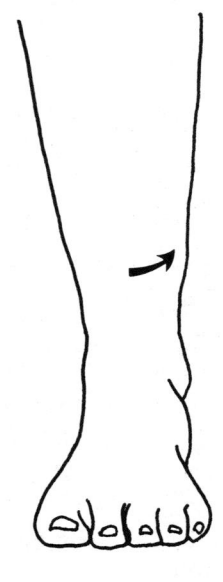

During midstance, external leg rotation is also occurring as it does during propulsion.

The difference between the two situations is that in the propulsive period, the heel is not on the ground, whereas it is on the ground during the midstance period.

The heel resists (by friction with the ground) the external rotation of the leg during midstance. However, during the propulsive period, the external leg rotation is only resisted by the friction of the forefoot against the ground. This causes the rearfoot to abduct on the forefoot as the leg externally rotates, or, put another way, the forefoot adducts on the rearfoot.

At the MTJ, the motions of plantarflexion and _____ are coupled as are the motions of dorsiflexion and _____.

adduction, abduction

13-66
So, when the forefoot adducts on the rearfoot during propulsion, it must also _____.

plantarflex

13-67
In this way, *the forefoot supinates around the MTJ o.a. during the propulsive period of gait.*

13-68
So, at the end of the propulsive period, around the MTJ l.a., the forefoot is in a _____ position while around the MT o.a., the forefoot is in a _____ position.

13: NORMAL MIDTARSAL JOINT FUNCTION IN THE GAIT CYCLE

pronated, supinated

13-69
From the following adjectives, pick those that describe the forefoot at the end of the propulsive period:

dorsiflexed/plantarflexed
inverted/everted
abducted/adducted

plantarflexed, everted, adducted

13-70
It is interesting that this is exactly opposite of the position that the foot started in at the beginning of the contact period.

13-71
During the contact period, the foot becomes a _____ _____ as the STJ _____.

mobile adaptor, pronates

13-72
At the same time, the MTJ l.a. is in a (*pronated/supinated*) position with the forefoot being _____ relative to the ground.

supinated, inverted

13-73
The forefoot is loaded during the _____ period from _____ to _____.

contact, lateral, medial

13-74
At the beginning of the contact period, the MTJ o.a. is in a _____ position because of the pull of the _____ _____ _____ and the _____ _____.

pronated, extensor digitorum longus, peroneus tertius

13-75
These muscles, along with the muscle which supinated the MTJ l.a. —the _____ _____—act to decelerate the plantarflexion of the foot just before and during the contact period.

anterior tibial

13-76
During the midstance period, the STJ _____.

supinates

13-77
Along with STJ supination is coupled _____ leg rotation.

external

13-78
The rearfoot is prevented from following the leg externally by friction with the ground.

As the STJ supinates during the midstance period, the MTJ l.a. (*pronates/supinates*) as the forefoot is stabilized by ground reaction forces.

pronates

13-79
During the midstance period, the MTJ o.a. remains in a _____ position.

pronated

13-80
Thus, at the end of the midstance period, i.e., _____ _____ of the same foot, both the MTJ l.a. and o.a. are in a _____ position.

heel lift, pronated

13-81
This combination of positions at the MTJ (i.e., with the forefoot pronated around both axes) allows normal propulsion to begin.

During the propulsive period, the MTJ l.a. remains in a _____ position so that the body weight may be shifted smoothly from _____ to _____.

pronated, lateral, medial

13-82
This shift of body weight is accomplished by use of the strong everters of the foot—the _____ muscles.

peroneal

13-83
During propulsion, since the heel is off of the ground, the rearfoot follows the leg as it _____ rotates.

Simultaneously, the STJ is _____.

externally, supinating

13-84
Since the forefoot is the only part of the foot in contact with the ground during the propulsive period, it resists the external rotation which the rearfoot is following.

The result is that the rearfoot is abducted on the forefoot, or, put another way, the forefoot is _____ on the rearfoot.

adducted

13-85
Adduction occurs around the MTJ _____ axis.

oblique

13-86
Coupled with adduction around the MTJ oblique axis is the motion of _____ _____.

plantarflexion

13-87
Actually, this makes very good sense. As the rearfoot follows the leg in external rotation, not only is it abducted away from the relatively stable forefoot, but it is also *dorsiflexed* relative to the forefoot.

13-88
So, during the propulsive period, the forefoot is in a _____ position around the MTJ o.a.

supinated

13-89
At the end of the propulsive period, the forefoot is then supinated around the MTJ o.a. and _____ around the MTJ l.a.

pronated

13-90
From the end of the propulsive period through about the middle of the swing phase, the forefoot stays pronated around the MTJ l.a. and *becomes* pronated around the MTJ o.a.

13-91
This follows since the STJ is also pronating for the same purpose—to shorten the effective length of the lower extremity so that it may clear the ground.

13-92
After the foot has cleared the ground, the forefoot progresses toward the position that it will be in at the beginning of the contact period— i.e., _____ around the MTJ o.a. and _____ around the MTJ l.a.

pronated, supinated

13-93
Congratulations! You have just completed the most conceptually difficult chapter in this book (so far)!

Questions

FRAME 13-7

1. During the stance period, MTJ *position* is controlled by:P
   a. STJ position
   b. gastrocnemius tension
   c. STJ motion
   d. forefoot reaction forces
   e. ground reaction forces

FRAME 13-14

2. During the *midstance* and *propulsive* periods, the available MTJ ROM:
   a. increases
   b. decreases
   c. stays the same
   d. increases, then decreases
   e. decreases, then increases

FRAMES 13-21 AND 13-22

3. Which of the following muscles will supinate the MTJ *longitudinal axis* when contracting?
   a. extensor digitorum longus
   b. anterior tibial
   c. peroneus tertius
   d. a and b
   e. a and c

FRAMES 13-29–13-31

4. At heel strike, the MTJ o.a. is in a pronated position while the MTJ l.a. is in a supinated position, causing the lateral aspect of the forefoot to come into contact with the ground first.
   a. true
   b. false

FRAME 13-39

5. The MTJ o.a. is maintained in a supinated position during the contact period of gait.
   a. true
   b. false

FRAME 13-31

6. Forefoot loading occurs from medial to lateral.
   a. true
   b. false

7. At the end of the midstance period, the forefoot is:
   a. pronated about the MTJ l.a. and supinated about the MTJ o.a.
   b. pronated about the MTJ l.a. and pronated about the MTJ o.a.
   c. supinated about the MTJ l.a. and pronated about the MTJ o.a.
   d. supinated about the MTJ l.a. and supinated about the MTJ o.a.
   e. none of the above

FRAMES 13-54—13-56

8. Throughout the propulsive period, the forefoot remains maximally supinated about the MTJ l.a.
   a. true
   b. false

FRAME 13-63

9. During the propulsive period, the:
   a. leg externally rotates
   b. forefoot abducts on the rearfoot
   c. forefoot adducts on the rearfoot
   d. a and b
   e. a and c

FRAME 13-65

10. In order for the propulsive period to begin, it is necessary that the forefoot be pronated about both of the MTJ axes.
    a. true
    b. false

FRAME 13-56

Answers

1. e
2. b
3. b
4. a
5. b
6. b
7. b
8. b
9. e
10. a

CHAPTER 14

Midtarsal Joint Deformity and Its Effects on the Gait Cycle

- forefoot varus—definition and etiology
- forefoot valgus—definition and etiology
- forefoot varus and valgus—relationship to MTJ range of motion
- forefoot supinatus—definition and etiology
- differentiating forefoot varus from forefoot supinatus
- compensation, signs, and symptoms of forefoot varus
- forefoot supinatus secondary to forefoot varus
- differentiating forefoot valgus from plantarflexed first ray
- compensation, signs, and symptoms of forefoot valgus

14-1
(Fig. 14.1) Recall that the index of MTJ position used clinically is the relationship between the plantar plane of the forefoot and the plantar plane of the rearfoot when the STJ is in its _____ position and the forefoot is maximally _____ around both of the MTJ axes.

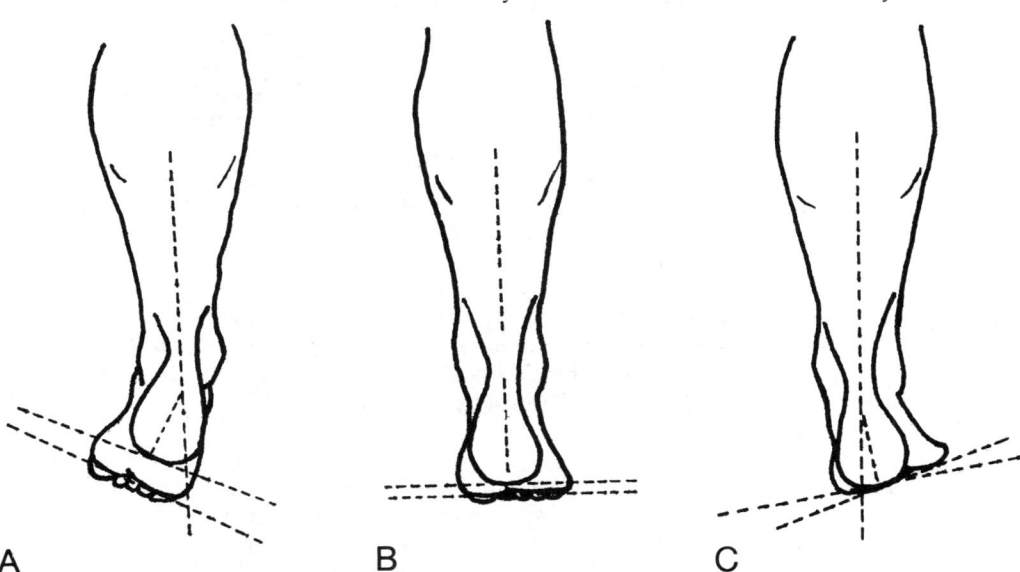

A   **B**   **C**

Figure 14.1 The STJ in its maximally pronated, neutral, and maximally supinated positions.

neutral, pronated

14-2
In the normal foot, with the STJ neutral and forefoot maximally pronated around both of the MTJ axes, the plantar plane of the forefoot would be (*inverted/parallel/everted*) relative to the plantar plane of the rearfoot.

parallel

14-3
Probably the two most common structural MTJ deformities are *forefoot varus* and *forefoot valgus*.

14-4
Forefoot varus refers to a structural abnormality in which the plantar plane of the forefoot is inverted relative to the plantar plane of the rearfoot when the STJ is in its neutral position and the forefoot is maximally pronated about both MTJ axes (Fig. 14.2).

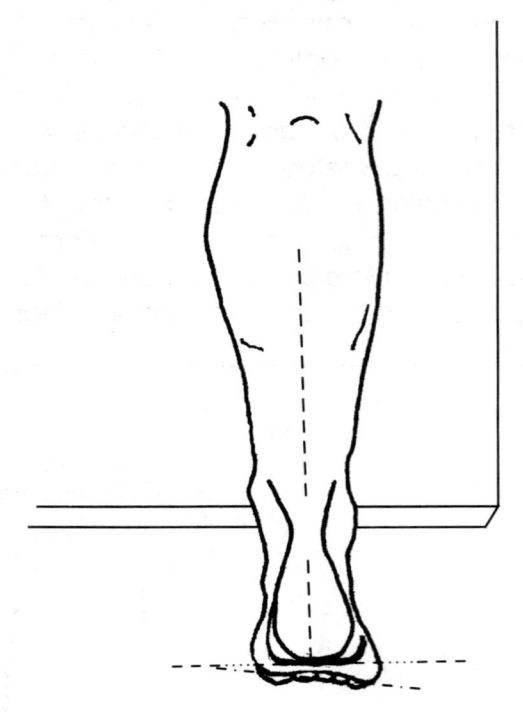

Figure 14.2.
Forefoot varus.

14-5
The two most common structural abnormalities of the MTJ are forefoot _____ and forefoot _____.

varus, valgus

14-6
Forefoot varus refers to the _____ abnormality in which the plantar plane of the forefoot is _____ relative to the plantar plane of the rearfoot with the STJ in its neutral position and the forefoot maximally pronated around both MTJ axes.

structural, inverted

14-7
The most common etiology of forefoot varus is failure (i.e., nonoccurrence or reduced occurrence) of the normal valgus torsion in the head and neck of the talus during gestation.

The normal valgus torsion of the talar head and neck is responsible for creating a frontal plane arch in the lesser tarsal bones with the concavity plantar (inferior). When this torsion fails to occur, the frontal plane arch does not appear either. As a result, the patient with this etiology of forefoot varus has a foot with a characteristically flat appearance of the dorsal aspect of the lesser tarsus (Fig. 14.3).

Additionally, the dorsal to plantar thickness in the area of the lesser tarsus is decreased.

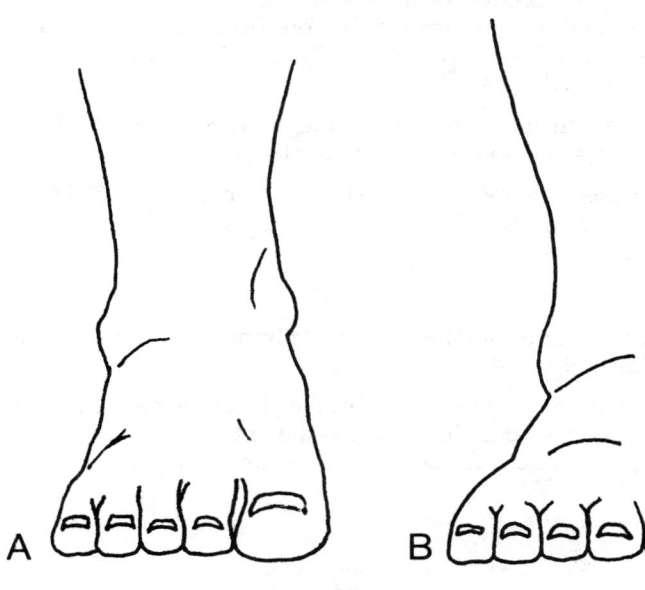

Figure 14.3.
A, A normal rectus foot. B, The forefoot varus foot exhibits a characteristic flattened appearance of the dorsal aspect of the lesser tarsus.

14-8
In a patient with forefoot varus, one would usually expect to see the lesser tarsus exhibit a(an) (*increased/unchanged/decreased*) dorsal to plantar thickness.

decreased

14-9
The most common etiology for forefoot varus is lack of the normal _____ torsion of the talar _____ and _____.

valgus, head, neck

14-10
As a result of this inadequate valgus torsion, the normal frontal plane arch observed in the lesser tarsus is (*increased/unchanged/decreased*).

decreased

14-11
This gives a characteristically _____ appearance to the dorsal aspect of the lesser tarsus.

flat

14-12
Another etiology of forefoot varus is a plantarflexed cuboid which, in turn, plantarflexes the fourth and fifth metatarsals relative to the first, second, and third metatarsals.

The interesting thing about this etiology of forefoot varus is that the flat appearance of the lesser tarsus and their decreased dorsal to plantar thickness *are both absent*.

A final etiology of forefoot varus is a plantarflexed fifth metatarsal which also establishes an inverted forefoot plane when compared with the rearfoot under standard conditions (STJ neutral and MTJ maximally pronated).

These points are mainly of academic note, however, since the functional status for all etiologies is essentially the same.

For our purposes, just recall that the most common etiology of forefoot varus is lack of normal _____ _____ of the talar _____ and _____.

valgus torsion, head, neck

14-13
The other relatively common *structural* deformity of the forefoot is forefoot valgus (Fig. 14.4).

As one might expect, in this condition, the plantar plane of the forefoot is _____ relative to the plantar plane of the rearfoot with the STJ in its _____ _____ and the MTJ maximally pronated.

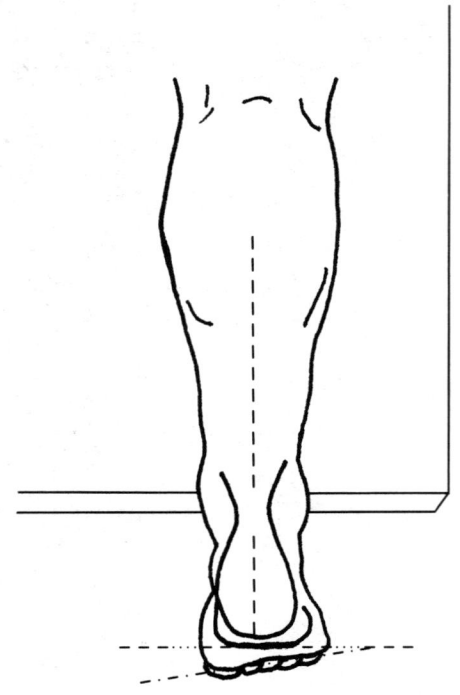

Figure 14.4.
Forefoot valgus.

14-14

everted, neutral position

Forefoot varus and forefoot valgus are the two most common _____ deformities of the MTJ.

14-15

structural

The plantar plane of the forefoot is everted relative to the plantar plane of the rearfoot (with the STJ neutral and the MTJ maximally pronated) in the structural deformity called _____ _____.

14-16

forefoot valgus

A very important clinical feature to remember about *forefoot valgus* is that *the first ray has a normal ROM.*

(There is a condition which will be discussed later in this chapter that is very similar to forefoot valgus but is differentiated in part by the first ray exhibiting an abnormal ROM.)

14-17

So, in the forefoot valgus, there is a _____ deformity of the MTJ in which the forefoot is _____ to the rearfoot and in which the first ray maintains a (*normal/abnormal*) ROM.

14-18

structural, everted, normal

Note that in a patient with forefoot valgus, the forefoot is *everted* relative to the rearfoot, but it is *not* abnormally pronated relative to the rearfoot.

Likewise, in the patient with forefoot varus, the forefoot is _____ relative to the rearfoot but is *not* abnormally supinated relative to the rearfoot.

14-19

inverted

This is a significant point of information since it illustrates that *forefoot varus and valgus deformities do not cause any alteration in the total ROM about the MTJ's two axes.*

Since these deformities are created by an osseous mechanism proximal (most of the time) or distal to the MTJ, the MTJ's total ROM is unchanged. That is to say, the MTJ is essentially normal in and of itself. The MTJ's orientation in space is the problem, secondary to the way the bones around it are holding it relative to the rest of the foot.

14-20

The MTJ total ROM in forefoot varus and forefoot valgus deformities is (*increased/unchanged/decreased*).

14-21

unchanged

In forefoot deformities which have soft tissue problems as their etiologies, one might expect the MTJ total ROM to be (*increased/unchanged/decreased*).

14-22

decreased

In fact, this is one of the clinical observations used to differentiate between a forefoot varus deformity and a forefoot supinatus deformity.

Forefoot supinatus is a relatively fixed, supinated position of the forefoot relative to the rearfoot caused by *soft tissue adaptation.*

14-23
In a patient with a forefoot supinatus deformity, one would expect to see a MTJ total ROM which is (*increased/unchanged/decreased*).

decreased

14-24
A forefoot supinatus deformity can be seen as a result of secondary soft tissue adaptation when a person walks with an everted calcaneus for a long enough time. (The calcaneus may be everted for a number of reasons ranging from congenital to compensatory.)

As the calcaneus is maintained in an everted position, the ground forces push the forefoot into a supinated position. This supinated position becomes more and more fixed as the soft tissues adapt into a contractured state about the MTJ.

This state of contracture causes the MTJ ROM to become decreased as contrasted with the osseous forefoot varus deformity in which the MTJ ROM is (*increased/unchanged/decreased*).

unchanged

14-25
These considerations are an important part of differentiating forefoot varus from forefoot supinatus deformities. The general principle of soft tissue etiologies causing restriction in a joint's ROM can also be applied to joints other than the MTJ.

14-26
Recall that in a forefoot varus deformity, with the STJ in its neutral position, the forefoot is inverted relative to the rearfoot (Fig. 14.5).

In forefoot varus, there is said to be *complete compensation* for this deformity *when the forefoot completely contacts the ground.*

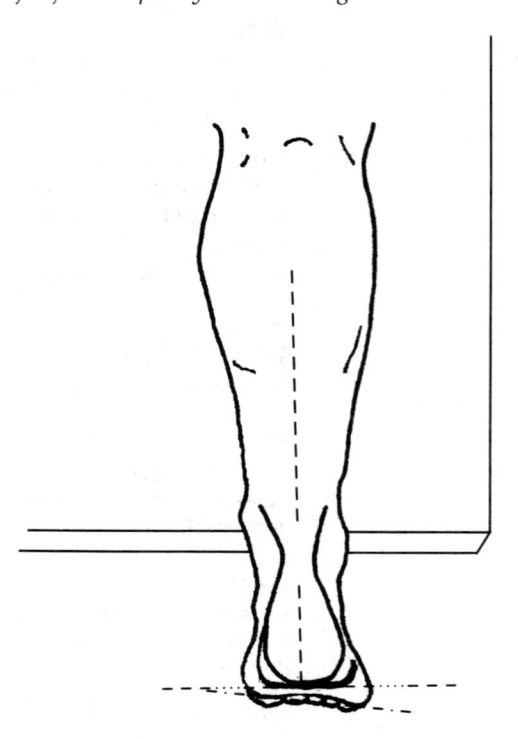

Figure 14.5.
Forefoot varus.

14-27
Complete the compensation of a forefoot varus deformity occurs when the _____ completely contacts the ground.

forefoot

14-28
This compensation is mainly a result of STJ pronation.

If there was no compensation by the STJ, the lateral aspect of the forefoot would be substantially overloaded during the weightbearing portion of the gait cycle, causing associated microtrauma with each step.

14-29
Forefoot varus is compensated for (mostly) by _____ _____.

STJ pronation

14-30
Additionally, there is some MTJ pronation which may occur to compensate for forefoot varus. More about this later.

14-31
If the amount of forefoot varus is 3° or less, the STJ will only compensate that specific number of degrees.

So, if a patient had a forefoot varus deformity of 2°, the STJ would pronate _____° only, in order to compensate that deformity.

2

14-32
If, however, the forefoot varus deformity is greater than 3°, the STJ will *maximally pronate* to the end of its ROM—i.e., it will pronate more than the number of degrees required to bring the forefoot's medial surface into contact with the ground.

14-33
So, the calcaneus will compensate only the specific number of degrees of deformity if the forefoot varus is _____° or less.

3

14-34
If the forefoot varus deformity is greater than 3°, the STJ will _____ _____.

maximally pronate

14-35
The reason that the STJ maximally pronates with a forefoot varus deformity of greater than _____° is that once the calcaneus is everted more than 3°, the force of the body's weight pushes it to the end of the STJ's pronatory ROM.

3

14-36
If, however, the STJ cannot completely compensate the forefoot varus deformity, then and only then will the MTJ pronate to help with the compensation. The MTJ pronation will occur mostly about its longitudinal axis.

14-37

Let's look at a few clinical examples to illustrate these various modes of compensation for forefoot varus.

Patient #1

Forefoot varus = 2°
STJ total ROM = 21°
No STJ deformity is present.

The STJ neutral position would be observed with the calcaneus vertical relative to the ground. There would be 7° of pronation available to the STJ from its neutral position. In order to compensate for the 2° forefoot varus deformity, the STJ would pronate 2° only. This would bring the forefoot into complete contact with the ground, thus completely compensating the forefoot varus deformity.

With the forefoot varus deformity completely compensated, the STJ would still have 5° of pronatory motion left which could be used as needed in the gait cycle.

14-38

Now you try one.

Patient #2

Forefoot varus = 4°
STJ total ROM = 21°
There is no STJ deformity present.

A) Calculate the position of the calcaneus (i.e., STJ) when compensation occurs for the forefoot varus deformity.

B) Is the compensation complete?

C) How much pronatory ROM is available to the STJ after it has compensated the forefoot varus deformity?

14-39

A) In Patient #2, since there is greater than 3° of forefoot varus, the STJ will pronate maximally to the end of its ROM.

B) The compensation is complete since the forefoot is now completely contacting the ground.

C) There is no pronatory ROM available to the STJ after it has functioned to compensate the forefoot varus since the STJ is maximally pronated to the end of its pronatory ROM.

14-40

Now, try this one.

Patient #3

Forefoot varus = 8°
STJ total ROM = 21°
There is no STJ deformity present.

A) Calculate the calcaneal (i.e., STJ) position once compensation has occurred for the forefoot varus deformity.

B) Is the STJ compensation complete?

C) How much pronatory ROM is available to the STJ after it has compensated the forefoot varus deformity?

D) Is MTJ compensation for the forefoot varus deformity involved in this case?

14-41

A) The calcaneal (i.e., STJ) position would be 7° everted since the STJ must maximally pronate to compensate forefoot varus deformities of greater than 3°.

B) The compensation by the STJ is not complete. The forefoot started 8° inverted to the rearfoot which was perpendicular to the ground. After the STJ maximally pronated, thus everting the forefoot along with it, the forefoot was still left 1° inverted relative to the ground. The STJ only had enough motion available to compensate 7° of the 8° of forefoot varus deformity.

C) After the compensatory function of the STJ has occurred, there is no further pronatory motion available to the STJ. It has maximally pronated to the end of its pronatory ROM in the process of compensating for the large forefoot varus deformity.

D) MTJ compensation for the forefoot varus deformity *is* involved in this case. In order to compensate for the 1° inverted position of the forefoot left after STJ compensation occurs, the MTJ pronates about its longitudinal axis to allow the forefoot to completely contact the ground.

14-42

It is interesting to note that a forefoot varus deformity which causes maximal STJ pronation can sometimes cause a forefoot supinatus deformity to develop.

Take an example where there is 4° of forefoot varus and 9° of STJ pronatory motion available. The first 4° of pronatory motion is all that is required to bring the medial aspect of the forefoot to the ground. However, since all of the STJ's pronatory ROM will be used up, the last 5° of pronatory STJ motion will jam the medial aspect of the forefoot into the ground, thus forcing it into an even more inverted position relative to the rearfoot than it was before any STJ compensation occurred.

When this type of compensation has occurred long enough, soft tissue adaptation will occur and an element of forefoot supinatus may be added to the pathologic complex.

14-43
So, to review, maximal STJ pronation occurs in order to compensate for _____° or more of forefoot varus.

3

14-44
The STJ will pronate only the same specific number of degrees as there is forefoot varus deformity if the forefoot varus deformity is less than or equal to _____°.

3

14-45
True or false: The MTJ will only help compensate for a forefoot varus deformity when that deformity is greater than the number of degrees of STJ pronatory motion available.

true

14-46
The effects of forefoot varus in gait vary with whether or not the deformity is *completely* compensated or only *partially* compensated.

However, in both completely and partially compensated forefoot varus cases, one thing is constant—the foot (and STJ) remain pronated throughout the entire stance phase of gait.

14-47

Since the STJ does not become supinated in the propulsive period of gait (Fig. 14.6), there is no stable platform available in the forefoot off of which the body weight can be propelled.

The result is an apropulsive gait in which the weightbearing foot with the deformity remains in contact with the ground longer in order to let the other foot establish a channel for the body weight which cannot be effectively propelled off of the unstable forefoot.

So, in both completely and partially compensated forefoot varus deformities, we would expect to see a STJ which is _____ throughout the stance phase of gait.

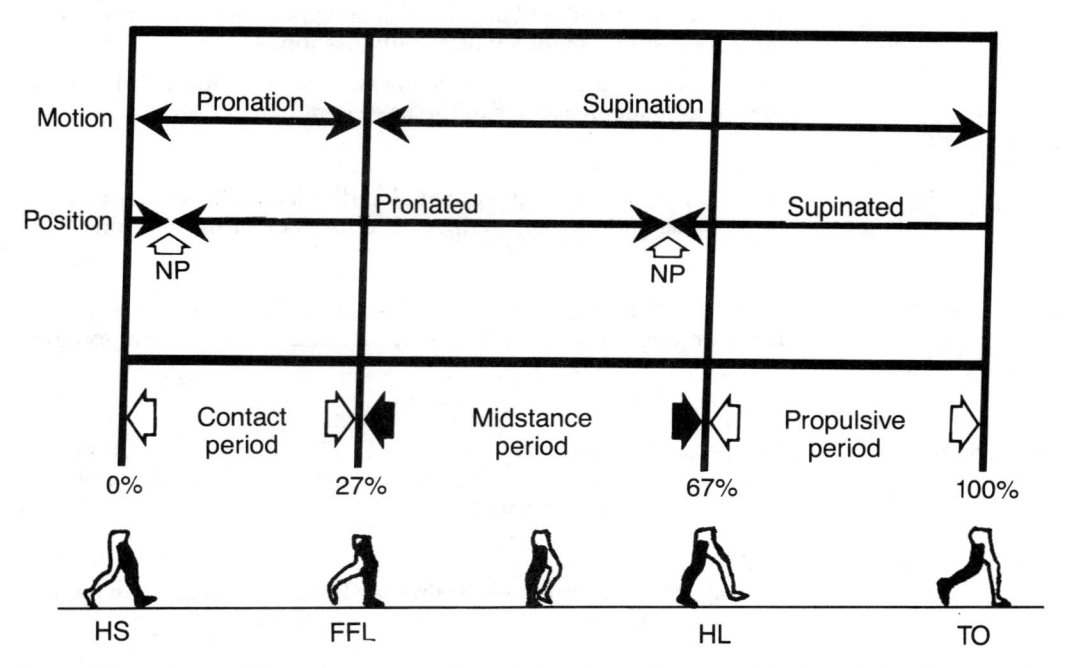

Figure 14.6. Normal STJ motion and position during the gait cycle. Note that during the propulsive phase, the STJ should normally be in a supinated position in order to provide a stable platform off of which to propel the weight.

pronated

14-48
The gait of a patient with forefoot varus would be (*propulsive/apropulsive*) when observed clinically.

apropulsive

14-49
This is because during the _____ period of the stance phase of gait, the forefoot cannot function as a stable platform from which body weight can be propelled.

propulsive

14-50
Additionally, one would expect to see muscle fatigue of the leg and foot since these muscles must overwork in a pronated foot to try and stabilize an unstable structure.

14-51
In the patient with partially compensated forefoot varus, the medial aspect of the forefoot (*is/is not*) contacting the ground.

is not

14-52
Since the STJ cannot get the medial aspect of the forefoot onto the ground, when the forefoot starts bearing significant weight during the midstance period, there is a weight overload on the lateral aspect of the foot. This ground force pushes the lateral aspect of the foot up in the direction of eversion. Since the lateral foot has no more eversion motion available to it—all STJ and MTJ motion in this direction has been used up—the body weight shifts medially in a frontal plane vector and causes the tibia to adduct at its proximal end, thus creating a momentary genu valgum configuration.

This periodic shift of tibial position can create a strain on both the medial and lateral aspects of the knee joint.

14-53
So, one possible etiology of medial and/or lateral knee strain would be a (*completely/partially*) compensated forefoot varus deformity.

partially

14-54
In fact, (especially) medial as well as lateral knee knee pain is seen not infrequently in patients with _____ compensated forefoot _____.

partially, varus

14-55
Muscle fatigue secondary to a _____ STJ position throughout the _____ phase of gait is observed in both partially and completely compensated forefoot varus.

pronated, stance

14-56
Medial and/or lateral knee strain may be seen in _____ compensated forefoot varus.

partially

14-57

Additionally, in *partially* compensated forefoot varus, hyperkeratotic accumulations may be seen at the plantar aspects of the *fourth and/or fifth* metatarsal heads (Fig. 14.7).

The reason for this callus distribution is that these two metatarsal heads receive a much higher than normal proportion of the body weight during the midstance and propulsive periods when the medial aspect of the foot would normally be sharing in weightbearing. Since the forefoot is maintained in an inverted position, the lateral metatarsals must bear an abnormally large amount of the body weight. This creates subcutaneous and dermal irritation superficial to the metatarsal head which leads to the formation of reactive hyperkeratosis.

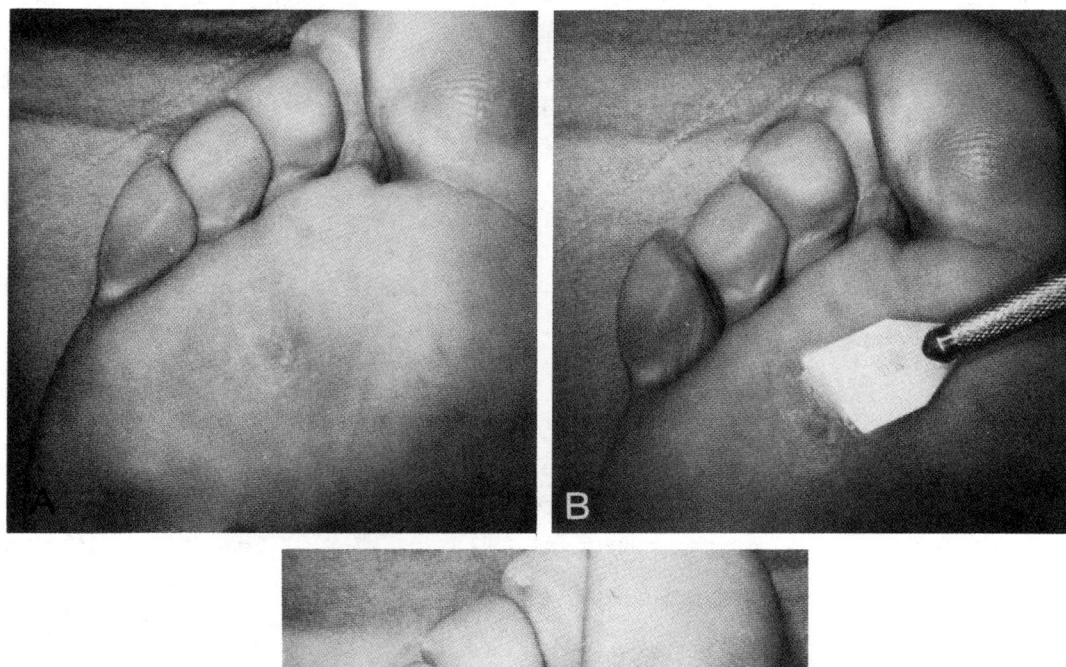

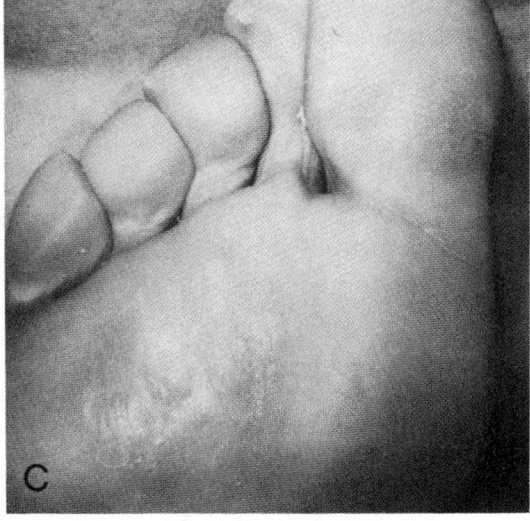

Figure 14.7. A callus beneath the fourth metatarsal head. (Reproduced with permission from Yale JF: *Yale's Podiatric Medicine,* ed 3. Baltimore, Williams & Wilkins, 1987, p 162.)

14-58
In partially compensated forefoot varus, calluses under the _____ and/or _____ metatarsal heads may be seen.

fourth, fifth

14-59
In contradistinction, the patient with a *completely* compensated forefoot varus may have a callus under the *second* metatarsal head (Fig. 14.8).

The reason for this is that in cases where a large amount of STJ pronatory motion exists in excess of that needed to compensate the forefoot varus deformity, the ground reactive forces push the medial side of the foot in the direction of supination (after the medial side contacts the ground). The first ray is able to get up out of the way since it has an independent axis of motion (relative to the second through fourth metatarsals). This leaves the second metatarsal head to receive the brunt of the ground reactive force pushing in a supinatory vector. The subsequent irritation superficial to the second metatarsal head causes the formation of the callus tissue.

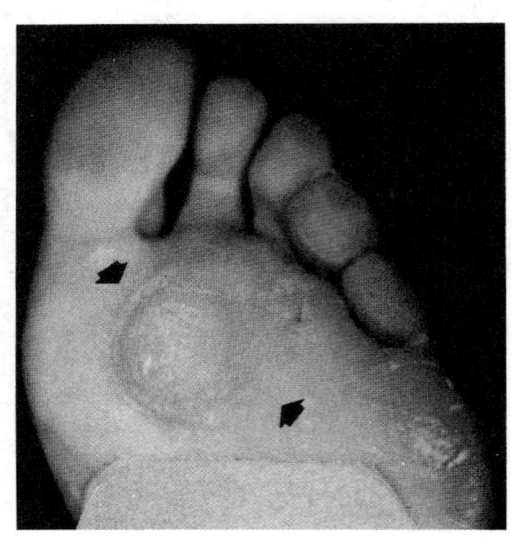

Figure 14.8.
A callus beneath the second metatarsal head. (Reproduced with permission from Yale JF: *Yale's Podiatric Medicine*, ed. 3. Baltimore, Williams & Wilkins, 1987, p 284.)

14-60
A callus may be seen under the fourth and/or fifth metatarsal heads in _____ compensated forefoot varus.

Calluses may be observed under the second metatarsal head in a patient with _____ compensated forefoot varus.

partially, completely

14-61
Medial and/or lateral knee strain may be encountered in the patient with _____ compensated forefoot varus.

partially

14-62
A clinical feature common in both partially and completely compensated forefoot varus is the presence of _____ _____ throughout the stance phase of gait.

14: MIDTARSAL JOINT DEFORMITY AND ITS EFFECTS ON THE GAIT CYCLE

STJ pronation

14-63
(Fig. 14.9) Consequently, other signs of excessive weightbearing STJ pronation may also be seen—Tailor's bunion, adductovarus hammertoe deformities of the fourth and fifth digits, hallux valgus deformity, as well as fatigue of the intrinsic and extrinsic muscles of the foot.

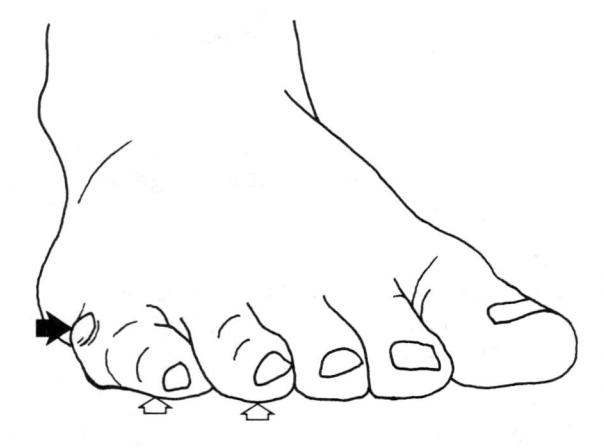

Figure 14.9. A tailor's bunion (solid arrow) and adductovarus contractures of the fourth and fifth digits (hollow arrowheads).

14-64
Recall that in forefoot varus, there is a(an) (*increased/unchanged/decreased*) dorsal to plantar thickness of the lesser tarsus.

decreased

14-65
The forefoot varus patient also has a (*flatter/rounder*) appearance to the dorsal aspect of the lesser tarsus.

flatter

14-66
The patient with only forefoot supinatus has neither of these findings. The lesser tarsus appear essentially normal.

14-67
In forefoot valgus, the plantar aspect of the forefoot is _____ relative to the plantar aspect of the rearfoot with the STJ in its neutral position and the MTJ maximally pronated.

everted

14-68
In the forefoot valgus deformity, the first ray has a normal range of motion.

In a plantarflexed first ray deformity, which will be covered later in Chapter 16, the first ray has an abnormal ROM.

Otherwise, the gross appearance of a forefoot valgus deformity and a plantarflexed first ray deformity is very similar.

14-69
Right now, the thing to remember is that in forefoot valgus, the first ray has a _____ range of motion.

normal

14-70
Since the forefoot is in an everted position in a forefoot valgus deformity, the compensation for this deformity is going to consist of measures which will _____ the forefoot back to the ground.

14-71
For the average MTJ axes and ROM, the *order* of compensation of forefoot valgus is first, the *longitudinal axis* of the MTJ, then supination of the *STJ*, then supination of the MTJ *oblique axis*, and, finally, further *STJ* supination. A helpful mnemonic for this order is: L.A.—S.O.S.

invert

14-72
So, the first joint axis about which forefoot valgus is compensated is the _____ _____ _____.

MTJ longitudinal axis

14-73
If this fails to adequately reduce the forefoot valgus by bringing the lateral aspect of the forefoot to the ground, the _____ joint will _____.

subtalar, supinate

14-74
If still more supination is required, it will come next from the _____ joint _____ axis; if even more is still needed, it will come from the _____ joint.

midtarsal, oblique, subtalar

14-75
If the forefoot valgus is competely compensated by supination of the MTJ longitudinal axis, the foot will appear normal in static stance.

The tipoff that a forefoot valgus deformity exists is that the fifth metatarsal head can be lifted from the ground without the calcaneus everting also. This is because there is some pronatory ROM available from the MTJ longitudinal axis since it has supinated to compensate for the everted forefoot position.

In a normal foot, lifting the fifth metatarsal head off of the ground will cause the calcaneus to evert simultaneously since there is no buffer of MTJ longitudinal axis motion available in the direction of pronation. Recall that in a normal foot the MTJ axes are both maximally pronated in the neutral and relaxed calcaneal stance positions.

14-76
So, if a forefoot valgus deformity can be completely compensated by MTJ longitudinal axis supination, the foot will appear (*normal/abnormal*).

normal

14-77
Once STJ supination is utilized to compensate for a forefoot valgus deformity, the foot will appear supinated in static stance.

14-78
At least superficially, it would seem that a forefoot valgus deformity compensated by MTJ longitudinal axis and STJ supination would look similar to an uncompensated rearfoot varus deformity.

In a cursory way, the two do look similar—both have a calcaneus with an inverted position. That is where the similarities end.

Keep in mind that uncompensated rearfoot varus describes a *maximally pronated* foot while the compensation for forefoot valgus involves *supination*.

14-79

In a pronated foot, one would expect to see the forefoot abducted on the rearfoot, a(an) (*increased/unchanged/decreased*) arch height, internal rotation of the leg, and the talus in an adducted position with its head prominent medially.

decreased

14-80

The supinated foot is just the opposite—a high-arched foot with the forefoot appearing adducted on the rearfoot, external rotation of the leg along with talar abduction, and no medial talar head prominence.

Remember that the tibia follows the talus in closed kinetic chain motion. When the talus abducts with STJ supination, the tibia rotates _____.

externally

14-81

So, the way to tell an STJ-compensated forefoot valgus from an uncompensated rearfoot varus is that the former will appear (*supinated/pronated*).

supinated

14-82

Recall that during the midstance period, the normal forefoot is progressively pronating about the MTJ longitudinal axis as the STJ supinates away from its contact period pronated position. In the normal foot, by the end of the midstance period when heel-off occurs, the MTJ is maximally pronated about both ot is axes, thus locking the forefoot against the rearfoot so that body weight can efficiently be transferred distally and medially into the forefoot.

Now picture what happens in the forefoot valgus foot that has required STJ supination for its compensation. During the first half of the midstance period, the foot remains supinated. *Towards the end of the midstance period, STJ pronation occurs.* This happens because if the foot's supinated attitude was maintained, the body weight could not be transferred medially in preparation for transfer to the contralateral foot.

14-83

So, in the STJ-compensated forefoot valgus, and at the end of midstance, the STJ is _____ instead of _____.

pronating, supinating

14-84

In order to keep the body weight medially, the STJ remains in a pronated position during most of the propulsive period, thus making the forefoot very unstable as a propulsive lever.

Finally, the foot necessarily supinates late in propulsion in order to allow transfer of body weight to the contralateral foot.

14-85

In the STJ-compensated forefoot valgus patient, since supination only occurs late in the _____ period, the patient's gait is *apropulsive*.

propulsive

14-86
The symptoms of forefoot valgus compensation are completely listed in Appendix 1. It is important to note that they vary with the levels of compensation required for the forefoot valgus.

One important contrast to be noted is that between the flexion contracture of the digits that occurs with MTJ longitudinal axis supination and the adducto-varus contracture that is seen with chronic pronation of the foot (Fig. 14.10).

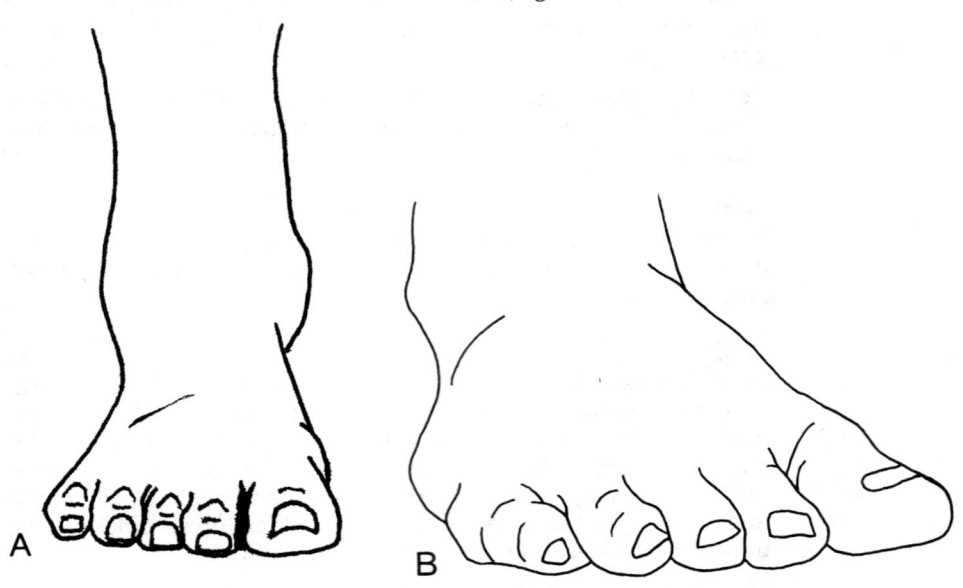

Figure 14.10. *A,* Flexion contractures of the digits may be seen with MTJ longitudinal axis supination. *B,* Adductovarus contractures of the fourth and fifth digits as may be seen with chronic pronation.

14-87
To compensate for forefoot valgus, there is first supination about the MTJ _____ axis.

longitudinal

14-88
As this supination occurs, the metatarsals may be carried into a plantarflexed attitude. (Some MTJ longitudinal axes permit more, and some less, of this sagittal plane motion to be coupled with the predominant frontal plane motions about that axis.)

As the metatarsals are carried into a plantarflexed position, they cause the proximal phalanges to become dorsiflexed. This increases the tension of the flexor tendons and causes the intermediate and distal phalanges to be pulled into a plantarflexed position.

Over time, this creates a *flexion contracture of the lesser digits.*

14-89
So, a flexion contracture of the lesser digits may be seen in a forefoot valgus which is compensated by MTJ _____ axis (*pronation/supination*).

14: MIDTARSAL JOINT DEFORMITY AND ITS EFFECTS ON THE GAIT CYCLE 183

14-90
Recall that with STJ pronation, the ability of the quadratus plantae to straighten out the flexor digitorum longus tendons is impaired. As a result, the vector of their pull changes from parallel and posterior to the phalanges to *medial* and posterior.

longitudinal, supination

The result of this is to create a deforming force on the lesser digits (most on the fifth and least on the second) towards the position of adduction and varus rotation. This creates the adductovarus type of contracture.

14-91
So, to review, in a forefoot valgus patient with compensation from MTJ longitudinal axis supination, a _____ type contracture of the lesser digits may be seen.

In a patient with chronic STJ pronation, the type of contracture of the lesser digits encountered is called _____.

14-92
Additionally, in the patient with MTJ longitudinal axis supinatory compensation for forefoot valgus, hyperkeratosis may be seen at the *plantar aspects of the first and fifth metatarsals.*

flexion, adductovarus

The first metatarsal bears the body weight much longer than usual because the abnormally everted position of the forefoot causes the first metatarsal to be the first part of the forefoot to receive weight as forefoot contact occurs. The weightbearing of this metatarsal continues throughout the rest of the stance phase of gait.

In addition to this excessive weightbearing irritation is the insult of the shearing force that occurs with supination of the MTJ longitudinal axis.

Together, these forces create substantial irritation which causes the reactive hyperkeratosis to occur beneath the first metatarsal head.

14-93
The fifth metatarsal head may have a callus at its plantar aspect because of the shearing force of compensatory supination. The middle three metatarsals are usually not involved because the inversion that occurs with the compensatory supination tends to keep the brunt of supinatory shearing limited to the first and fifth metatarsals.

14-94
To review, in the forefoot valgus patient with compensatory MTJ longitudinal axis supination, a _____ contracture of the _____ digits may be observed.

14-95
Also, a callus may be seen at the plantar aspects of the _____ and _____ metatarsals.

flexion, lesser

14-96
Additionally, lateral knee strain may be seen in the forefoot valgus patient because of the quick STJ pronation that occurs just prior to the end of the propulsive period.

first, fifth

14-97

In this chapter, we have covered three of the most common MTJ abnormalities encountered clinically: forefoot varus, forefoot valgus, and forefoot supinatus.

There are other abnormalities (e.g., plantarflexed first ray) which affect MTJ biomechanics, but these are not primary problems of the MTJ, and are covered in Chapter 16.

Questions

FRAMES 14-4 AND 14-22

1. A *structural* deformity of the MTJ in which the plantar plane of the forefoot is inverted relative to the plantar plane of the rearfoot, when the STJ is in its neutral position and the forefoot is maximally pronated about both MTJ axes, is called:
   a. forefoot valgus
   b. forefoot supinatus
   c. forefoot varus
   d. a and b
   e. b and c

FRAME 14-7

2. The *most common* etiology of forefoot varus is:
   a. failure of the normal valgus torsion of the calcaneus during gestation
   b. failure of the normal varus torsion of the calcaneus during gestation
   c. excessively pronated position of the rearfoot during gestation
   d. failure of the normal varus torsion of the talar head and neck during gestation
   e. failure of the normal valgus torsion of the talar head and neck during gestation

FRAME 14-16

3. In the patient forefoot valgus, one would expect to find a normal first ray ROM.
   a. true
   b. false

FRAMES 14-18 AND 14-19

4. In the patient with forefoot valgus, the forefoot is:
   a. inverted relative to the rearfoot
   b. supinated relative to the rearfoot
   c. everted relative to the rearfoot
   d. pronated relative to the rearfoot
   e. none of the above is correct

5. Soft tissue adaptation is the etiology for:
   a. rearfoot varus
   b. rearfoot valgus
   c. forefoot varus
   d. forefoot valgus
   e. forefoot supinatus

FRAME 14-22

6. *Complete* compensation of a forefoot varus deformity occurs when the:
   a. forefoot first contacts the ground
   b. forefoot completely contacts the ground
   c. forefoot propels effectively off of the ground
   d. rearfoot reaches perpendicular to the ground
   e. rearfoot does not pronate during the propulsive period

FRAME 14-26

7. If a forefoot varus deformity is measured to be 4°, one would expect the compensatory mechanism to include maximal STJ pronation.
   a. true
   b. false

FRAMES 14-31 AND 14-32

8. The thing that distinguishes *completely* compensated forefoot varus from *partially* compensated forefoot varus is that only in the latter do the foot and STJ remain pronated throughout the entire stance phase of gait.
   a. true
   b. false

FRAMES 14-46 AND 14-47

9. In patients with partially compensated forefoot varus, it is not uncommon to observe:
   a. foot and leg fatigue
   b. medial knee strain
   c. lateral knee strain
   d. a and b
   e. a, b, and c

FRAMES 14-50–14-52

10. In the STJ-compensated forefoot valgus patient, supination occurs late in the propulsive period, thus rendering the patient's gait apropulsive.
    a. true
    b. false

FRAMES 14-84 AND 14-85

Answers

1. c
2. e
3. a
4. c
5. e
6. b
7. a
8. b
9. e
10. a

CHAPTER 15

Function of the First and Fifth Rays and the Metatarsophalangeal Joints

- review of first ray axis and motion
- relationship of STJ position and first ray motion
- abnormal STJ pronation and first ray hypermobility
- first ray hypermobility as an etiology of hallux abductovalgus and hallux limitus/rigidus
- first ray motion and position in the gait cycle
- review of fifth ray axis and motion
- digital function in gait

15-1
Before discussing the function of the first ray, let's review its normal axis and motion. Recall that the axis of the first ray is practically parallel to a transverse plane (Fig. 15.1). This means that the first ray (*will/will not*) exhibit motion in the transverse plane.

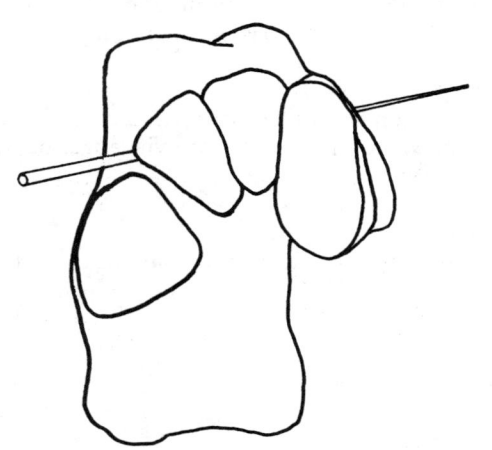

Figure 15.1.
A distal view of the axis of the first ray. Note that it is almost parallel to a transverse plane.

15-2
will not
First ray motion may, however, be observed in the _____ and _____ planes in roughly equal amounts (i.e., 1:1).

15-3
frontal, sagittal
The reason that motion in the frontal and sagittal planes is roughly equal is that the axis of the first ray is angulated about 45° from each of these two planes (Fig. 15.2).

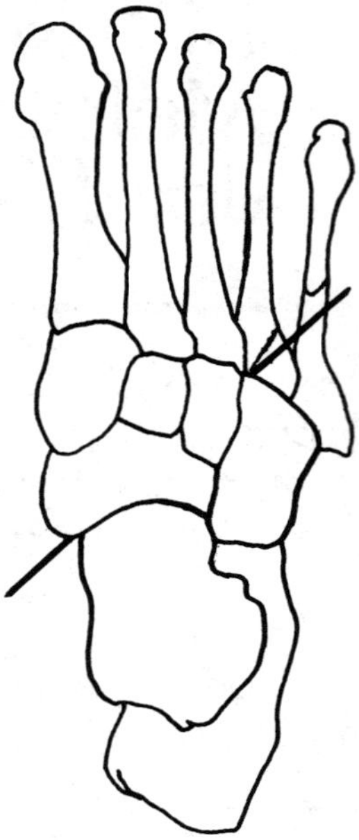

Figure 15.2.
A dorsal view of the first ray's axis.

15-4
So, one would expect just as much dorsiflexion-plantarflexion to be available about the axis of the first ray as there is _____-_____.

15-5
inversion-eversion
Recall that there is a coupling of motion in the _____ and _____ planes about the axis of the first ray.

15-6
frontal, sagittal
Inversion is coupled with _____. (HINT: Look at the orientation of the axis of the first ray and visualize the motion which would occur about it.)

15-7
dorsiflexion
The converse is also true; plantarflexion is coupled with _____.

15: FUNCTION OF THE FIRST AND FIFTH RAYS AND THE METATARSOPHALANGEAL JOINTS

15-8
(Fig. 15.3. See the preceding frames.)

eversion

Recall that, like the MTJ, the motion of the first ray is linked to the position of the STJ. Like the MTJ, the first ray has an *increased* range of motion (ROM) when the STJ is in a (pronated/neutral/supinated) position.

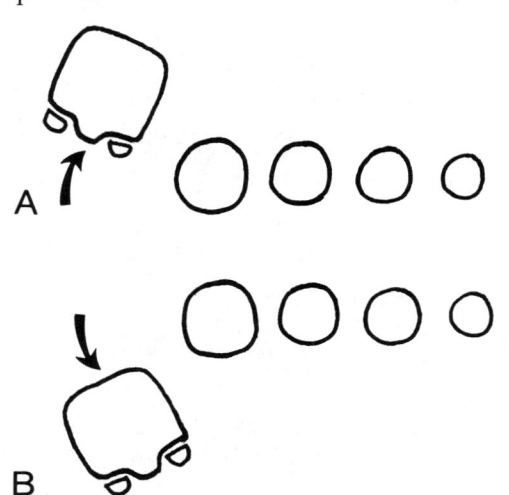

Figure 15.3.
A, With first ray dorsiflexion, simultaneous inversion occurs. B, With plantarflexion of the first ray, simultaneous eversion occurs.

15-9

pronated

Conversely, the first ray is most rigid (i.e., has the smallest ROM) when the STJ is in a (pronated/neutral/supinated) position.

15-10
(Fig. 15.4. See frames 15-8 and 15-9.)

supinated

Functionally, this works well in the normal foot, since during propulsion it is necessary for the first ray to be rigid in order to help propel the body weight. During propulsion, the STJ is (*pronating/supinating*).

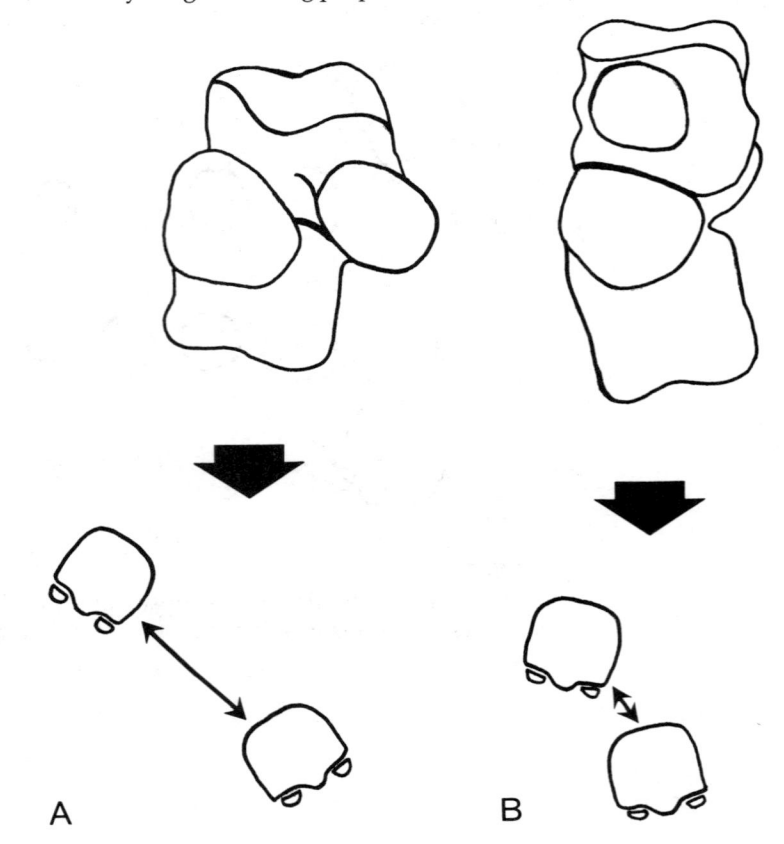

Figure 15.4.
A, Maximum STJ pronation causes an increase in the first ray range of motion. *B*, STJ supination causes a decrease in the range of motion available for the first ray.

supinating

15-11
In an abnormal situation, the STJ will pronate during the propulsive period (Fig. 15.5). This causes the first ray to become unstable and unable to function well as a weight bearing segment.

This situation is called *hypermobility of the first ray* and occurs with STJ pronation during the propulsive period of gait.

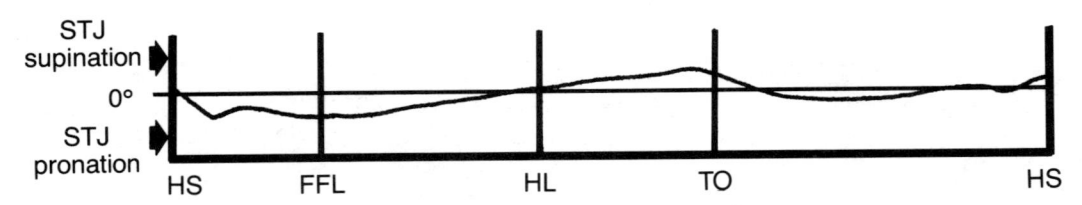

Figure 15.5. Normally during the propulsive period, the STJ is supinating which allows first ray stability.

15-12
When STJ pronation during propulsion causes instability of the first ray as a weightbearing segment, it is called _____ of the first ray.

hypermobility

15-13
This hypermobility causes subluxation of the first metatarsophalangeal joint (MPJ) which can, in turn, lead to deformity at that joint.

The first MPJ deformities which may occur as the result of a hypermobile first ray (secondary to _____ of the STJ during the propulsive period) are *hallux abductovalgus* and *hallux limitus/hallux rigidus* (Fig. 15.6).

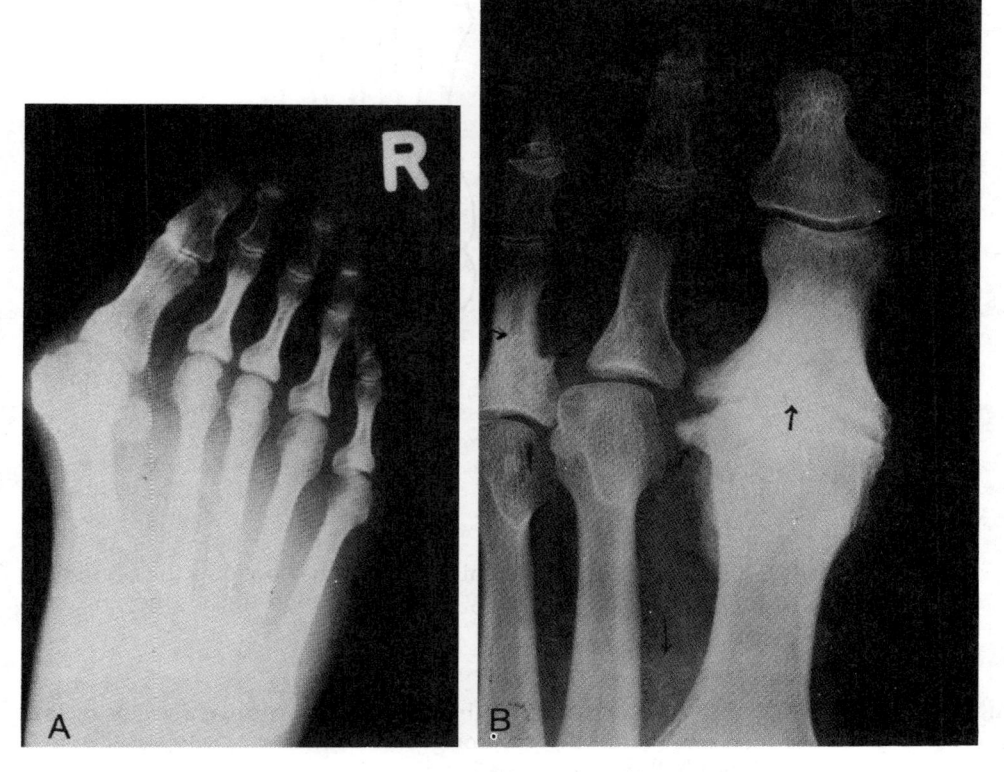

Figure 15.6. *A*, X-ray of a patient with hallux abductovalgus. *B*, X-ray of a patient with hallux limitus. (Reproduced with permission from Yale JF: *Yale's Podiatric Medicine*. ed. 3. Baltimore, Williams & Wilkins, 1987, p 399 and 350.)

pronation

15-14
Whether hallux limitus/hallux rigidus or hallux valgus occurs is the result of the primary vector of subluxation at the first MPJ.

If the primary vector of subluxation at the first MPJ is in the *transverse plane* (Fig. 15.7), as occurs in a *forefoot adductus* foot type, the *hallux abductovalgus* deformity will prevail.

Figure 15.7.
The solid arrow illustrates the transverse plane vector of subluxatory force that occurs in a forefoot adductus foot type when there is propulsive period STJ pronation. This is one of the etiologic factors in the development of a hallux abductovalgus deformity.

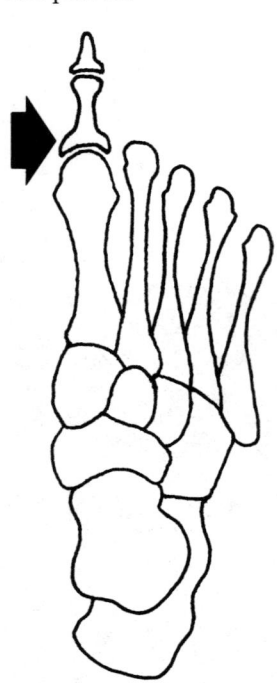

15-15
Hallux valgus and hallux limitus/rigidus may occur as the result of a _____ first ray, secondary to STJ pronation during the _____ period of gait.

hypermobile,
propulsive

15-16
If the resultant first MPJ subluxation has its primary vector in the transverse plane, the deformity most likely to develop at the first MPJ is a hallux _____ deformity.

abductovalgus

15-17
The foot type which predisposes to the development of first MPJ (predominantly) transverse plane subluxation is a (*forefoot rectus/forefoot adductus*) foot type.

15: FUNCTION OF THE FIRST AND FIFTH RAYS AND THE METATARSOPHALANGEAL JOINTS

forefoot adductus

15-18
The hallux limitus/rigidus deformity is more likely to develop in a patient with a forefoot rectus type of foot, where the primary subluxatory vector is in the sagittal plane (Fig. 15.8).

This sagittal plane subluxation causes the first MPJ to be jammed at its dorsal aspect during the propulsive period.

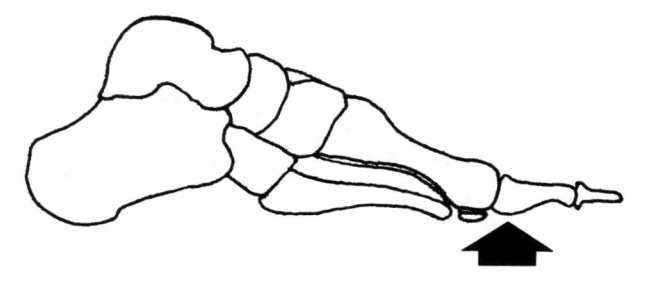

Figure 15.8. With propulsive period STJ pronation in a rectus type foot, the first MPJ subluxatory force occurs in a sagittal vector (solid arrow), thus predisposing to the development of a hallux limitus/hallux rigidus deformity.

15-19
When hypermobility of the first ray is the etiology of hallux abductovalgus, the most likely foot type for the patient to have is the forefoot _____ foot type.

If the patient has hallux limitus or rigidus, the most likely accompanying foot type is the forefoot _____ foot type.

adductus, rectus

15-20
In the patient with hallux limitus or rigidus, the primary subluxatory vector of force is in the _____ plane.

In the patient with hallux abductovalgus, the primary subluxatory vector is in the _____ plane.

sagittal, transverse

15-21
To get back to the *normal* situation, there is coupling of first ray plantarflexion with _____. There seems to be functional integration of these two motions in the propulsive period of gait.

eversion

15-22
We know that during propulsion, the foot prepares to propel the body weight and transfer it to the other foot.

The body weight ends up at the distal aspect of the first ray toward the end of the propulsive period. Since the foot is moving to achieve a slightly supinated attitude just before toe off, it is necessary for the first ray to be able to plantarflex in order to maintain weightbearing ability (i.e., in order to keep the medial aspect of the foot in contact with the ground).

In order that the tibial and fibular sesamoids be used as a stable foundation for the first metatarsal head, the motion of eversion is coupled with that of plantarflexion.

By keeping the first metatarsal weightbearing and stable against the sesamoids, the first metatarsal is able to function as a solid foundation against which the hallux may be stabilized in order to receive the body weight during propulsion.

15-23
So, during the propulsive period of gait, in order for the first ray to maintain weightbearing capability, the first ray must be able to _____ and _____.

plantarflex, evert

15-24
During the contact period, the STJ is (*pronating/supinating*).

pronating

15-25
This STJ pronation during the contact period (*increases/does not change/decreases*) the first ray's ROM.

increases

15-26
This allows the forefoot to be more flexible and better able to adapt for variances in terrain early in the stance phase of gait.

15-27
So, during the contact period, STJ pronation makes the whole foot (including the first ray) more of a (*mobile adaptor/rigid lever*).

mobile adaptor

15-28
In terms of actual *motion* of the first ray, it would be correct to say that it *starts late in the midstance period and continues on until late in the propulsive period.*

15-29
It is worthwhile to note that during the swing phase, the first ray is held in a dorsiflexed position.

15-30
To review the first ray, it has motion available in the _____ and _____ planes.

frontal, sagittal

15-31
Inversion is coupled with _____, and eversion is coupled with _____.

15: FUNCTION OF THE FIRST AND FIFTH RAYS AND THE METATARSOPHALANGEAL JOINTS

dorsiflexion, plantarflexion

15-32
Motion of the first ray begins late in the _____ period and ends late in the _____ period.

midstance, propulsive

15-33
This motion consists of _____ coupled with _____.

plantarflexion, eversion

15-34
These motions allow the _____ aspect of the foot to stay in contact with the ground and allow the first metatarsal to serve as a stable foundation so that the _____ can receive the body weight.

medial, hallux

15-35
Toward the end of the propulsive period, the first ray is in a (*dorsiflexed/plantarflexed*) position.

During the swing phase, the first ray is held in a (*dorsiflexed/plantarflexed*) position.

plantarflexed, dorsiflexed

15-36
STJ pronation during the propulsive period causes _____ of the first ray to occur.

hypermobility

15-37
With hypermobility of the first ray, if the primary subluxatory vector at the first MPJ is in the sagittal plane, the resulting deformity will be hallux _____.

limitus/rigidus

15-38
Hallux limitus usually occurs in a forefoot (*rectus/adductus*) type of foot.

rectus

15-39
In the patient that develops hallux abductovalgus as the result of hypermobility of the first ray, one would expect to find a forefoot (*rectus/adductus*) foot type with the predominant subluxatory vector being in the _____ plane.

adductus, transverse

15-40
To review the fifth ray axis and motion, recall that the axis runs in the same spatial orientation as that of the STJ—(dentist's degree) _____, _____, and _____ to proximal, lateral, and plantar.

15-41
(Fig. 15.9.)

distal, medial, dorsal

The motion that occurs about the fifth ray axis is (*monoplane/biplane/triplane*) motion—i.e., _____ and _____.

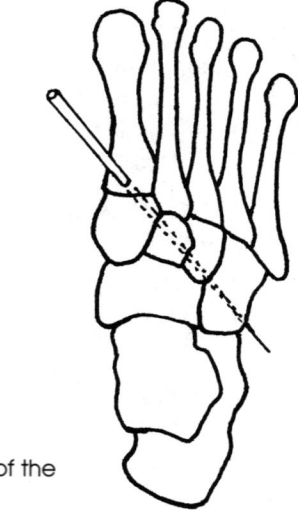

Figure 15.9.
A dorsal view of the fifth ray axis.

15-42

triplane, pronation, supination

While the axis and motion of the fifth ray are known, its function in gait is not well defined.

15: FUNCTION OF THE FIRST AND FIFTH RAYS AND THE METATARSOPHALANGEAL JOINTS

15-43
Recall that the metatarsophalangeal joints (MPJs) have axes (Fig. 15.10) which share a common spatial orientation with the axes of the interphalangeal joints (IPJs) and the central three rays.

All of these axes rest parallel to the frontal and transverse planes. This means that motion is only available in the _____ plane.

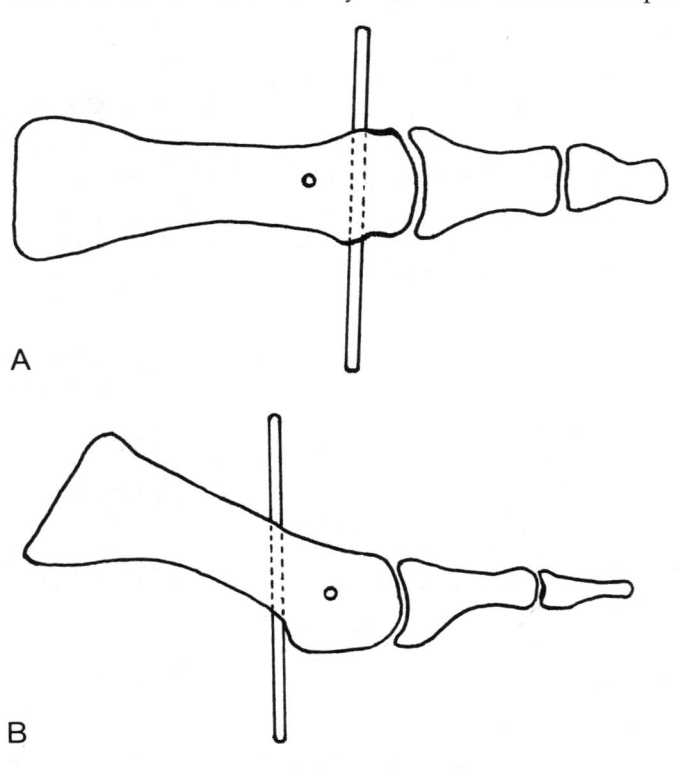

Figure 15.10.
A, A dorsal view of the MPJ axes. B, A lateral view of the MPJ axes.

sagittal

15-44
So, the toes can only move in the directions of either _____ or _____.

dorsiflexion, plantar-flexion

15-45
The toes only bear weight during one of the three periods of the stance phase of gait. Can you guess which one it would be?

propulsive period

15-46
In fact, during the propulsive period, the toes are undergoing *dorsiflexion* at the MPJs.

15-47
The toes are stabilized as a weightbearing platform by the *flexor digitorum longus* muscle. As a result, the body weight can be effectively propelled off of this platform toward the other foot.

15-48
To review, the toes undergo which motion during the propulsive period of gait?

dorsiflexion

15-49
The toes are stabilized as a weightbearing platform by the _____ _____ _____ muscle.

flexor digitorum longus

15-50
With the toes functioning as a stable platform, body weight can be effectively propelled to the opposite foot.

When the toes are functional as a stable platform for this purpose, it is called a *propulsive* gait.

Conversely, if the toes for some reason cannot function as a stable platform for the propulsion of weight to the opposite foot, the gait is called *apropulsive*.

15-51
So, when the toes cannot function as a stable platform from which to propel the body weight toward the opposite foot, the gait is called _____.

apropulsive

15-52
This concludes the chapter. The following chapter will use your foundation of knowledge regarding the first ray in order to examine and understand first ray pathology and the effect that it may have on the gait cycle.

Questions

1. The first ray does *not* clinically exhibit motion in the:
    a. sagittal plane
    b. transverse plane
    c. frontal plane
    d. a and b
    e. b and c

FRAME 15-1

2. In the examination of first ray motion, one would note that inversion is coupled with:
    a. abduction
    b. adduction
    c. dorsiflexion
    d. plantarflexion
    e. none of the above is correct

FRAMES 15-6 AND 15-7

15: FUNCTION OF THE FIRST AND FIFTH RAYS AND THE METATARSOPHALANGEAL JOINTS 199

FRAMES 15-8 AND 15-9

3. The first ray has a decreased ROM when the STJ is in a pronated position.
   a. true
   b. false

FRAMES 15-10–15-13

4. STJ pronation during the propulsive period of gait causes:
   a. hypermobility of the first ray
   b. first MPJ subluxation
   c. flexion deformity of the lesser digits
   d. a and b
   e. b and c

FRAME 15-14

5. When hypermobility of the first ray exists and a secondary hallux abductovalgus deformity develops, the patient probably has a:
   a. forefoot rectus foot type
   b. predominant vector of subluxation in the sagittal plane
   c. forefoot adductus foot type
   d. a and b
   e. b and c

FRAME 15-18

6. A patient that has hallux limitus secondary to propulsive STJ pronation and first ray hypermobility has the primary vector of subluxation in the:
   a. sagittal plane
   b. transverse plane
   c. frontal plane
   d. a and b
   e. b and c

FRAME 15-22

7. During the propulsive period, in order to have weightbearing integrity, the first ray must be able to plantarflex and evert.
   a. true
   b. false

FRAME 15-45

8. Joints with axes which rest parallel to the frontal and transverse planes include the:
   a. MPJs
   b. IPJs
   c. first ray
   d. a and b
   e. b and c

FRAME 15-46

9. During the propulsive period, the toes exhibit:
   a. inversion
   b. eversion
   c. plantarflexion
   d. dorsiflexion
   e. supination

FRAME 15-50

10. When the toes are functional as a stable platform during the propulsive period:
    a. it is called a propulsive gait
    b. body weight cannot be effectively transferred to the opposite foot
    c. it is called an apropulsive gait
    d. a and b
    e. b and c

Answers

1. b
2. c
3. b
4. d
5. c
6. a
7. a
8. d
9. d
10. a

CHAPTER
16

First Ray Pathology and Its Effect on the Gait Cycle

- plantarflexed first ray—definition and clinical recognition
- differentiating plantarflexed first ray from forefoot valgus
- effects of plantarflexed first ray on other foot joints
- effects of plantarflexed first ray in the gait cycle
- compensation for plantarflexed first ray
- metatarsus primus elevatus—definition and clinical recognition
- effects of metatarsus primus elevatus on other foot joints
- effects of metatarsus primus elevatus in the gait cycle
- effects of first ray pathology on the muscles of the leg

16-1
The first ray serves an important weightbearing function during the _____ period of the stance phase of gait.

propulsive

16-2
Naturally, anything which would compromise this weightbearing function could impair the foot's propulsive capability.

One first ray deformity which can do this is called *plantarflexed first ray*.

This is defined as a *structural* abnormality in which the first ray has *more plantarflexion than dorsiflexion* (Fig. 16.1). This is observed as the first metatarsal head is moved in relation to the plane of the second through fifth metatarsal heads, with the STJ in its neutral position and the MTJ completely pronated.

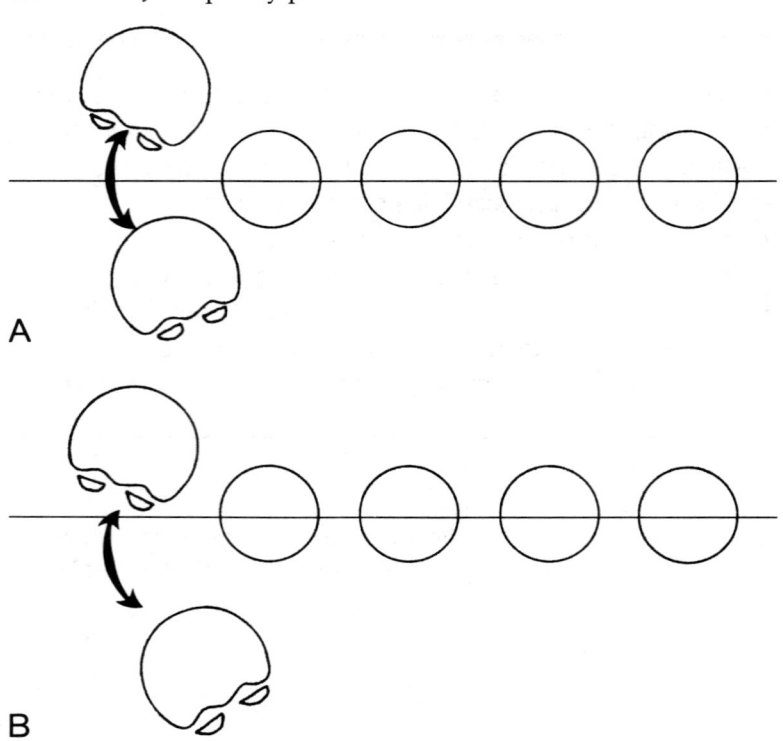

Figure 16.1.
A, The normal first ray range of motion. B, In a plantarflexed first ray deformity, the first ray has more plantarflexion than dorsiflexion available.

16-3
A plantarflexed first ray is similar to forefoot valgus, except that in forefoot valgus, the first ray has a (*normal/abnormal*) range of motion (ROM).

16-4

normal

(Fig. 16.2 See the above frame.)

In a plantarflexed first ray deformity, the first ray has an abnormal ROM in that there is more (*plantarflexion/dorsiflexion*) available than there is (*plantarflexion/dorsiflexion*).

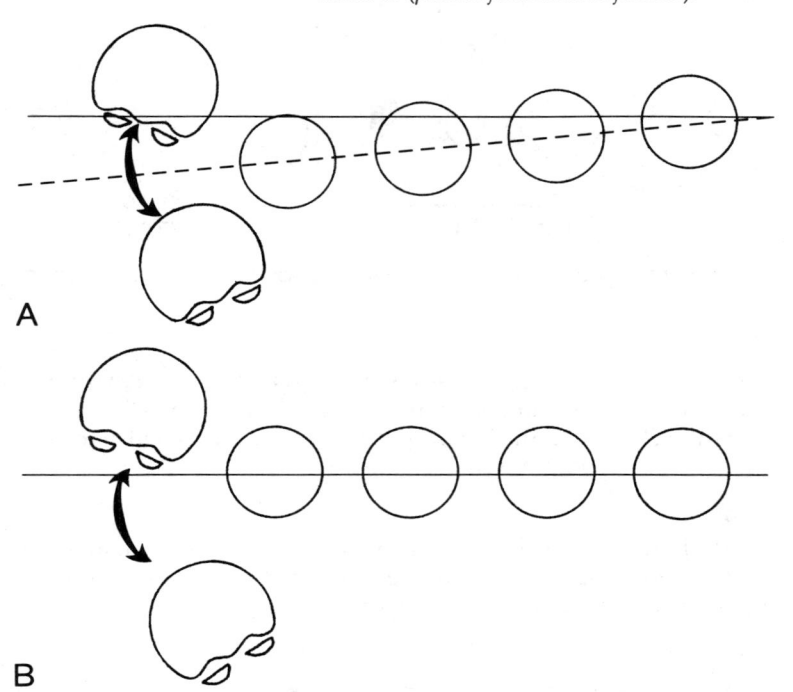

Figure 16.2.
A, Forefoot valgus. Note that the first ray has a normal range of motion. B, In a plantarflexed first ray deformity, the first ray has an abnormal range of motion.

16-5

plantarflexion, dorsiflexion

The gross morphology of a plantarflexed first ray mimics that of a forefoot valgus deformity—the plantar plane of the forefoot appears _____ relative to the plantar plane of the rearfoot with the STJ neutral and the MTJ maximally pronated.

16-6

everted

Additionally, the mechanisms of compensation for forefoot valgus and plantarflexed first ray deformities are similar.

Recall that in a forefoot valgus deformity, during propulsion the STJ is forced to (*pronate/supinate*) in order to keep the body weight medial in the foot.

pronate

16-7
This creates instability in the foot in general but, specifically, at the MTJ and the in the first ray.

The plantarflexed first ray deformity causes the same type of compensation to occur (Fig. 16.3).

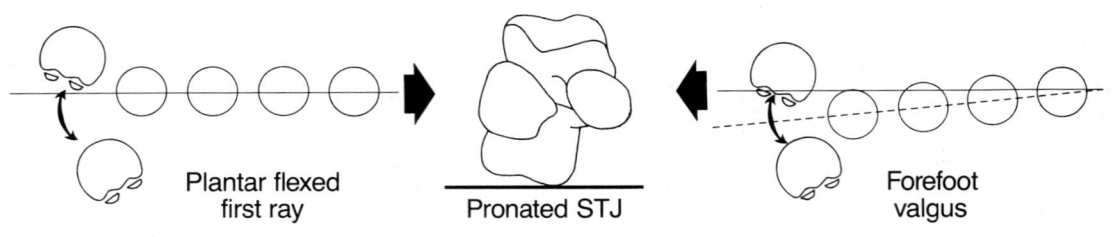

Figure 16.3. STJ pronation is the common method of compensation for both plantarflexed first ray and forefoot valgus.

Plantar flexed first ray — Pronated STJ — Forefoot valgus

16-8
So, in both plantarflexed first ray and forefoot valgus deformities, one would expect to find the forefoot _____ relative to the rearfoot and the STJ _____ during the propulsive period instead of the normal _____ motion.

everted, pronating, supinatory

16-9
The STJ pronation that occurs in both deformities serves to make the first ray very unstable, thus rendering it ineffective as a weightbearing platform and weight transfer conduit.

16-10
In a plantarflexed first ray deformity, since the first ray is made unstable during the _____ period by STJ _____, it cannot function as a secure foundation against which the hallux can stabilize itself to receive the body weight (in addition to the first ray having a poor capacity to *transmit* body weight).

propulsive, pronation

16-11
Not only is the first MPJ thus made unstable, but secondary to STJ pronation, the lesser digit MPJs are rendered unstable. (The forefoot is not adequately locked against the rearfoot and the long flexor pull is vectored *medial* and proximal instead of just proximal.)

In these ways, a plantarflexed first ray deformity (as well as a _____ _____ deformity) render the gait apropulsive.

forefoot valgus

16-12
Anytime that there is an apropulsive gait, a great deal of excess energy is required by the muscles of the lower extremity as they try to stabilize an unstable structure. (Some estimates run as high as 300% more utilization of energy with an unstable foot vs. a stable foot!)

16: FIRST RAY PATHOLOGY AND ITS EFFECT ON THE GAIT CYCLE

16-13
In plantarflexed first ray and forefoot valgus deformities, during propulsion (when the STJ is _____ to keep the medial aspect of the foot on the ground), the MTJ is supinating about its longitudinal axis to try and get the lateral aspect of the foot into contact with the ground.

Normally, the MTJ is maximally pronated about its longitudinal axis during propulsion so that the peroneus longus muscle can pull up the lateral side of the foot, effecting a lateral to medial transfer of weight.

In the plantarflexed first ray or forefoot valgus type of foot, since the MTJ is *not* maximally pronated about its longitudinal axis during propulsion, the weight transfer from medial to lateral is much more difficult to accomplish.

pronating

16-14
So, the effects of a plantarflexed first ray deformity on the biomechanics of the propulsive period are substantial.

Because of first ray instability (i.e., hypermobility), there is difficulty in achieving the normal weightbearing function of that segment.

The hypermobility of the first and lesser MPJs causes the gait to be _____.

apropulsive

16-15
This same hypermobility causes a much higher expenditure of _____ as the muscles work to try and stabilize the foot.

energy

16-16
In the plantarflexed first ray deformity, the hallux (*does/does not*) serve as a stable weight receptive segment.

does not

16-17
The reason for this is that since the first ray is not stable, the hallux has nothing solid against which it can stabilize itself to receive weight.

16-18
The order of joint compensation is the same in plantarflexed first ray and forefoot valgus deformities. The mnemonic for this is _____-_____.

L.A.-S.O.S.

16-19
This means that the first specific joint and axis around which compensation for a plantarflexed first ray deformity occurs is the _____ _____ axis.

MTJ longitudinal

16-20
If the plantarflexed first ray deformity is not completely compensated for by motion about the MTJ longitudinal axis, the next thing to occur is (*pronation/supination*) about the _____ joint.

supination, subtalar

16-21
If this fails to completely compensate the plantarflexed first ray deformity, then there will be supination of the MTJ _____ axis and, if needed, further compensation via more supination about the _____ joint.

oblique, subtalar

16-22
Another deformity of the first ray which will affect the propulsive period of gait is called *metatarsus primus elevatus*.

This is defined as a *structural* abnormality of the first ray in which the first ray has *more dorsiflexion than plantarflexion* (Fig. 16.4). This again is relative to the plane of the second through the fifth metatarsal and is defined with the STJ in its neutral position and the MTJ maximally pronated about both of its axes.

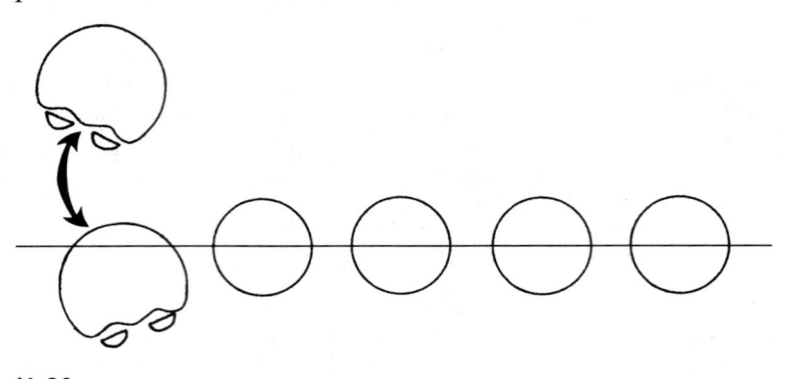

Figure 16.4.
Metatarsus primus elevatus. Note that the first ray has more dorsiflexion than plantarflexion available.

16-23
More plantarflexion than dorsiflexion is found in a _____ _____ _____ _____ deformity.

plantarflexed first ray

16-24
More dorsiflexion than plantarflexion is found in a _____ _____ _____ deformity.

16: FIRST RAY PATHOLOGY AND ITS EFFECT ON THE GAIT CYCLE

metatarsus primus elevatus

16-25
Clinically, in metatarsus primus elevatus, the first metatarsal head will be prominent at the dorsal aspect of the foot (Fig. 16.5).

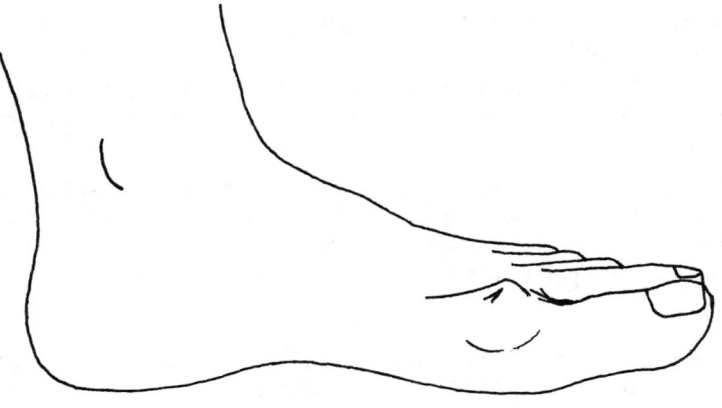

Figure 16.5. Metatarsus primus elevatus frequently demonstrates a dorsal prominence at the area of the first metatarsal head.

16-26
A first ray deformity which looks very similar to forefoot valgus is called _____ _____ _____.

plantarflexed first ray

16-27
A deformity of the first ray in which the first metatarsal head is prominent dorsally is called _____ _____ _____.

metatarsus primus elevatus

16-28
In metatarsus primus elevatus, there is more (*plantarflexion/dorsiflexion*) than (*plantarflexion/dorsiflexion*).

dorsiflexion, plantarflexion

16-29
As you might guess, a patient with metatarsus primus elevatus has a problem utilizing the first ray as a weightbearing segment during the late midstance and the propulsive periods.

Since it is in a relatively dorsiflexed position, there is difficulty in getting it down to the ground in order to bear weight.

16-30
In metatarsus primus elevatus, the first ray is in a relatively _____ position. As a result, there is difficulty in utilizing it as a weightbearing segment during the late _____ and _____ periods.

dorsiflexed, midstance, propulsive

16-31
Since the first ray is not stable during the propulsive period, the hallux has no secure foundation against which to stabilize itself.

Additionally, the STJ must sacrifice its optimal supinated position during the propulsive period to try and get the medial aspect of the foot down to the ground.

In the patient with metatarsus primus elevatus, during the propulsive period, the STJ is either slightly pronated or at its neutral position.

Since the STJ is not supinated, the MPJs are not well stabilized by the long flexors. The hallux is not very functional as a weight-receptive/weightbearing segment. These factors cause a relatively apropulsive gait in the patient with metatarsus primus elevatus.

16-32
So, in both plantarflexed first ray and metatarsus primus elevatus deformities, there is a (*propulsive/apropulsive*) gait.

apropulsive

16-33
One difference between the two deformities, however, is that in a metatarsus primus elevatus deformity, there is excessive weightbearing force exerted on the second metatarsal head both during the midstance and propulsive periods.

This causes a reactive hyperkeratosis to develop plantar to the second metatarsal head in the patient with metatarsus primus elevatus (Fig. 16.6).

Figure 16.6.
Calluses beneath the second metatarsal head may be seen in patients with metatarsus primus elevatus. (Reproduced with permission from Yale JF: *Yale's Podiatric Medicine,* ed. 3. Baltimore, Williams & Wilkins, 1987, p 284.)

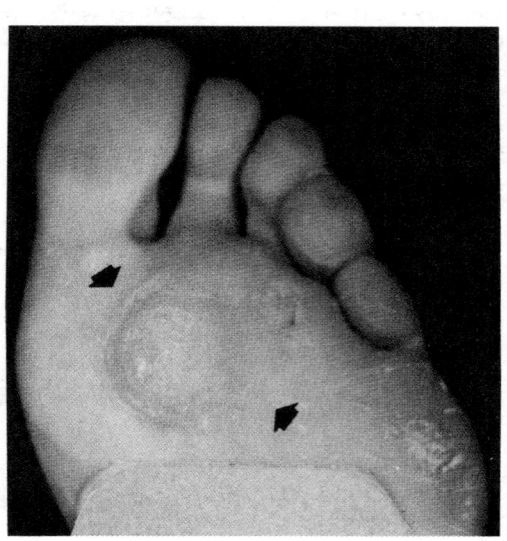

16-34
The patient with metatarsus primus elevatus has a first ray held in a relatively _____ position.

16-35

dorsiflexed

Some clinical signs of a patient with metatarsus primus elevatus are a first metatarsal head which is prominent at the _____ aspect of the foot, an _____ gait, and a callus plantar to the _____ metatarsal head.

16-36

dorsal, apropulsive, second

The reason for the callus plantar to the second metatarsal head in metatarsus primus elevatus is the weight overload which is borne there during the _____ and _____ periods of the stance phase of gait.

16-37

midstance, propulsive

In both plantarflexed first ray and metatarsus primus elevatus deformities, the foot is relatively unstable during the propulsive period. This makes the muscles of the foot and leg work much harder to stabilize the foot, thus producing *muscle fatigue* as an associated symptom of both deformities.

16-38

In metatarsus primus elevatus, since the first ray is held in a relatively _____ position, the hallux is forced into a relatively plantarflexed position. The hallux range of dorsiflexion is thus limited, and *repeated attempts at propulsion without adequate hallux dorsiflexion can secondarily produce a hallux limitus or hallux rigidus deformity.*

16-39

dorsiflexed

Recall that the primary subluxatory vector in patients with hallux limitus is in the _____ plane.

16-40

(Fig. 16.7. Refer to the above frame.)

sagittal

The (*dorsal/plantar*) aspect of the first MPJ becomes jammed since there is inadequate hallux (*dorsiflexion/plantarflexion*).

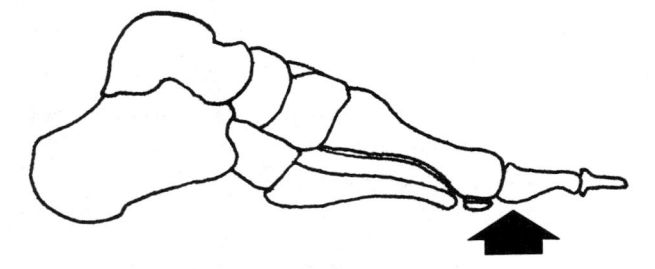

Figure 16.7. Patients with hallux limitus may have had subluxatory forces in the sagittal plane.

dorsal, dorsiflexion	**16-41** So, in a patient with metatarsus primus elevatus, one would expect to see associated _____ of the muscles of the leg and foot, as well as possibly a secondary hallux _____ or hallux _____ deformity.
fatigue, limitus, rigidus	**16-42** Hallux limitus and rigidus can occur in patients with metatarsus primus elevatus because the hallux has inadequate (*dorsiflexion/plantarflexion*) during the _____ period.
dorsiflexion, propulsive	**16-43** Another condition of the first ray which can cause a hallux limitus or rigidus deformity is *hypermobility*. While hypermobility of the first ray is not a deformity of the first ray, it is a condition which occurs secondary to STJ _____ during the _____ period of gait.
pronation, propulsive	**16-44** When hallux limitus or rigidus occurs as the result of first ray hypermobility, the foot type usually associated with it is the forefoot (*rectus/adductus*) type of foot.
rectus	**16-45** This ends the chapter on first ray pathology. The next two chapters deal with various aspects of the biomechanical examination and should help to further integrate some of the knowledge that you have gained.

Questions

FRAME 16-2

1. A *structural* abnormality in which the first ray has *more plantarflexion than dorsiflexion* is called:
   a. metatarsus primus varus
   b. metatarsus primus valgus
   c. metatarsus primus elevatus
   d. plantarflexed first ray
   e. dorsiflexed first ray

FRAME 16-5

2. Forefoot valgus differs from a plantarflexed first ray deformity in that patients with forefoot valgus have a normal first ray ROM whereas patients with plantarflexed first ray deformities do not.
   a. true
   b. false

FRAMES 16-6–16-9

3. STJ pronation during the propulsive phase, which causes the first ray to be ineffective as a weightbearing platform and weight-transfer conduit, occurs in both forefoot valgus and plantarflexed first ray.
   a. true
   b. false

FRAMES 16-6–16-13

4. In a plantarflexed first ray deformity, during propulsion, the:
   a. MTJ is pronating about its longitudinal axis
   b. STJ is pronating
   c. MTJ is supinating about its longitudinal axis
   d. a and b
   e. b and c

FRAME 16-19

5. The first specific joint axis about which compensation occurs for a plantarflexed first ray deformity is the:
   a. MTJ oblique axis
   b. STJ
   c. MTJ longitudinal axis
   d. a and b
   e. b and c

FRAME 16-22

6. Metatarsus primus elevatus is defined as a deformity in which:
   a. the hallux is not weight receptive
   b. the subluxatory vector at the first MPJ is in the sagittal plane
   c. the first ray has more plantarflexion than dorsiflexion
   d. the first ray has more dorsiflexion than plantarflexion
   e. the first ray has a normal ROM

FRAME 16-25

7. The first metatarsal head will be prominent at the dorsal aspect of the foot in:
   a. forefoot varus
   b. forefoot valgus
   c. metatarsus primus elevatus
   d. metatarsus primus varus
   e. plantarflexed first ray

FRAME 16-31

8. In the patient with metatarsus primus elevatus:
   a. the STJ is slightly supinated during the propulsive period
   b. the MPJs are well stabilized by the flexors during the propulsive period
   c. the hallux is functional as a weightbearing segment during the propulsive period
   d. the gait is relatively apropulsive
   e. the first ray is reasonably stable during the propulsive period

FRAMES 16-31 AND 16-32

9. In metatarsus primus elevatus, unlike a plantarflexed first ray deformity, there is a relatively apropulsive gait.
   a. true
   b. false

FRAME 16-33

10. In metatarsus primus elevatus, unlike a plantarflexed first ray deformity, there is excessive weightbearing force exerted on the second metatarsal head.
    a. true
    b. false

Answers

1. d
2. a
3. a
4. e
5. c
6. d
7. c
8. d
9. b
10. a

CHAPTER

17

Biomechanical Examination: Non-weightbearing Assessment

- normal ankle joint dorsiflexion and its measurement
- definition and clinical recognition of ankle equinus
- definition and clinical recognition of soleus equinus
- definition and clinical recognition of gastrocnemius equinus
- STJ measurements and neutral position calculation
- MTJ measurements
- first ray measurements
- malleolar torsion

17-1
The biomechanical examination will integrate much of the information that you have learned from the preceding chapters.

If there are any areas which are unclear to you, it may help if you go back to the appropriate chapter for a quick review.

17-2
In performing the non-weightbearing (NWB) portion of the biomechanical examination, it is necessary to keep two principles in mind:

A) In most patients, morphology and range of motion are symmetrical or close to it.

B) NWB findings must be correlated with findings from the rest of the biomechanical examination.

17-3
It is (*important/redundant*) to compare findings and measurements between the right and left sides in the NWB examination.

important

17-4

In the biomechanical examination, there are certain so-called "criteria for normalcy" (see Appendix 2) that reflect the ideal biomechanical parameters in the foot and lower extremity.

These ideal relationships seldom exist clinically.

They represent that which is ideal and, consequently, that which serves as the standard against which we evaluate.

17-5

The first measurement taken is that of *ankle dorsiflexion*. It is taken with the patient in the supine position.

Recall that inadequate ankle joint dorsiflexion can cause abnormal STJ pronation during the propulsive period of gait.

17-6

The minimum ankle dorsiflexion that is necessary for normal ambulation to occur is 10° with the knee extended (Fig. 17.1).

If a patient has less than 10° of ankle dorsiflexion with the knee extended (i.e., an "equinus" state), they may have abnormal STJ _____ occurring during the _____ period of gait.

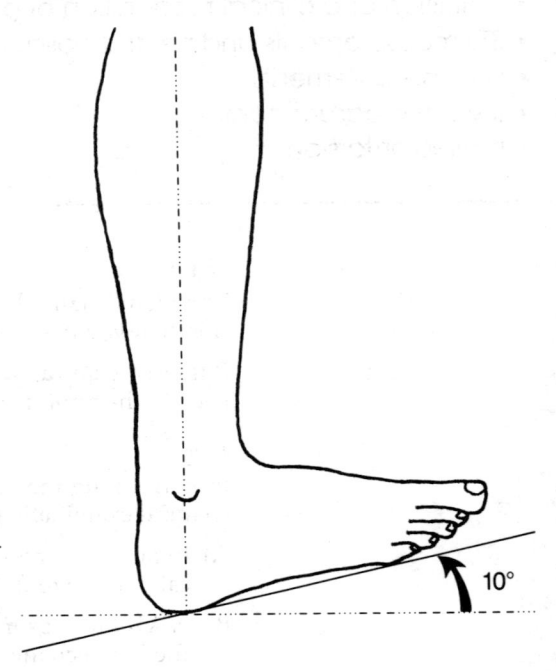

Figure 17.1.
The minimum amount of ankle joint dorsiflexion with the knee extended necessary for normal ambulation is 10°.

17: BIOMECHANICAL EXAMINATION: NON-WEIGHTBEARING ASSESSMENT 215

pronation, propulsive

17-7
We also measure the ankle dorsiflexion with the knee in a flexed position (Fig. 17.2). This is especially important when an equinus state exists (i.e., less than _____° of dorsiflexion available at the ankle).

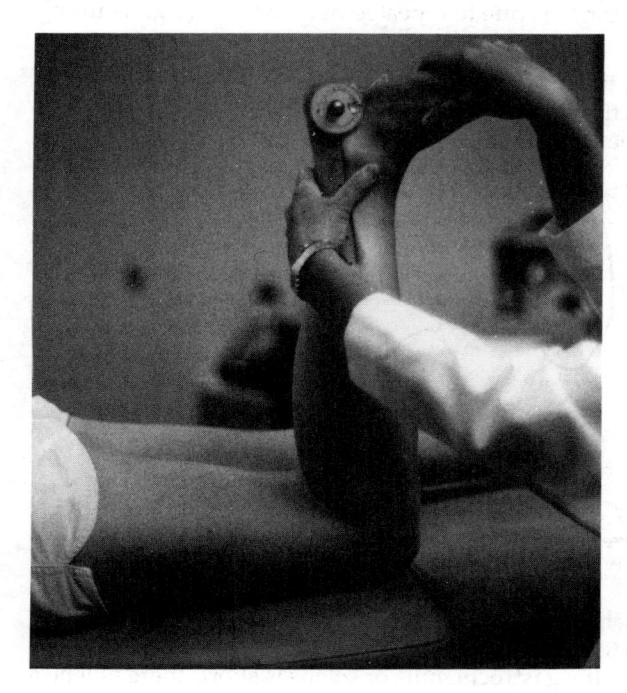

Figure 17.2.
Ankle joint dorsiflexion is also measured with the knee flexed.

10

17-8
Since flexing the knee relaxes the gastrocnemius muscle, there should be (*more/less*) dorsiflexion available at the ankle with the knee flexed.

more

17-9
If the amount of ankle dorsiflexion is the same with the knee extended and flexed, we know that the thing stopping the ankle at its end of dorsiflexion cannot be the _____ muscle.

The two most likely etiologies for equinus under these circumstances would be ankle equinus and soleus equinus (i.e., shortening or contracture of the soleus muscle).

17-10

"Ankle equinus" refers to a restriction of ankle joint dorsiflexion of less than _____° (with the knee extended) due to a bony blocking of motion, usually at the anterior ankle joint (Fig. 17.3). Frequently the osseous "lipping" is due to repeated microtrauma (e.g., running up hills).

Remember that in both ankle equinus and soleus equinus, there is the same restriction of ankle joint dorsiflexion present with the knee extended and flexed.

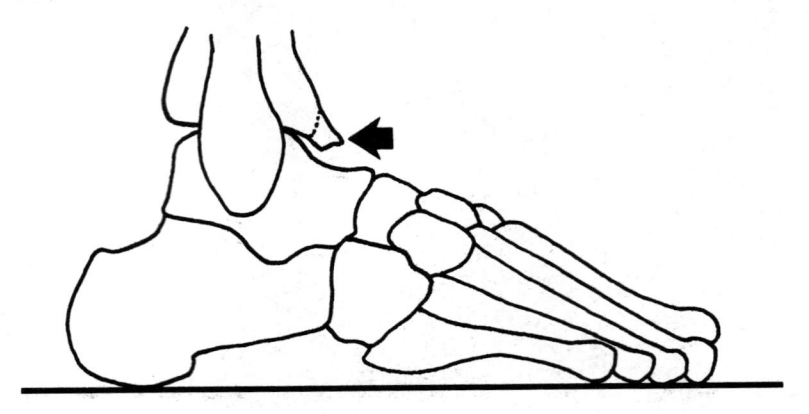

gastrocnemius

Figure 17.3.
A bony block at the anterior tibia can cause an ankle equinus.

10

17-11

Recall from anatomy that the tendon of the soleus joins that of the gastrocnemius to form the Achilles tendon which inserts into the calcaneus. If either the gastrocnemius or soleus is short, there will be a restriction of dorsiflexion at the ankle joint.

The same restriction of dorsiflexion will be present with both the knee extended and flexed if the muscle that is short is the _____.

soleus

17-12

A shortened gastrocnemius, on the other hand, will cause a restriction of ankle joint dorsiflexion that is greater with the knee _____ than it is with the knee _____. This is called a gastrocnemius equinus.

extended, flexed

17-13

The reason for this is that when the knee is flexed, the gastrocnemius muscle is relatively (*relaxed/tightened*), thereby permitting greater dorsiflexion at the ankle joint.

relaxed

17-14

To review, the two types of equinus that will cause an equal restriction of dorsiflexion at the ankle with the knee flexed and extended are _____ equinus and _____ equinus.

17: BIOMECHANICAL EXAMINATION: NON-WEIGHTBEARING ASSESSMENT 217

ankle, soleus

17-15
The type of equinus that causes a greater restriction of dorsiflexion with the knee extended than with it flexed is a _____ equinus.

gastrocnemius

17-16
Ankle joint dorsiflexion is measured with the patient in the _____ position and with the knee _____ and _____.

supine (or sitting), flexed, extended

17-17
In order for normal ambulation to occur, there should be at least _____° of dorsiflexion available at the ankle joint with the knee _____.

10, extended

17-18
If less than 10° of dorsiflexion is available to the ankle joint, there will probably be abnormal STJ _____ during the _____ period of gait.

pronation, propulsive

17-19
Another measurement that is taken in the NWB examination is that of the *STJ total ROM* so that the *neutral position* can be calculated.

The posterior aspect of the calcaneus is bisected, as is the posterior aspect of the distal one-third of the leg.

Since the posterior surface of the calcaneus is rotated slightly from the frontal plane, it is necessary—before making the bisections—to bring it into a frontal plane. This is accomplished by having the patient flex their opposite knee and hip (Fig. 17.4), thus elevating the pelvis on that side and rotating the lower extremity on the side being examined.

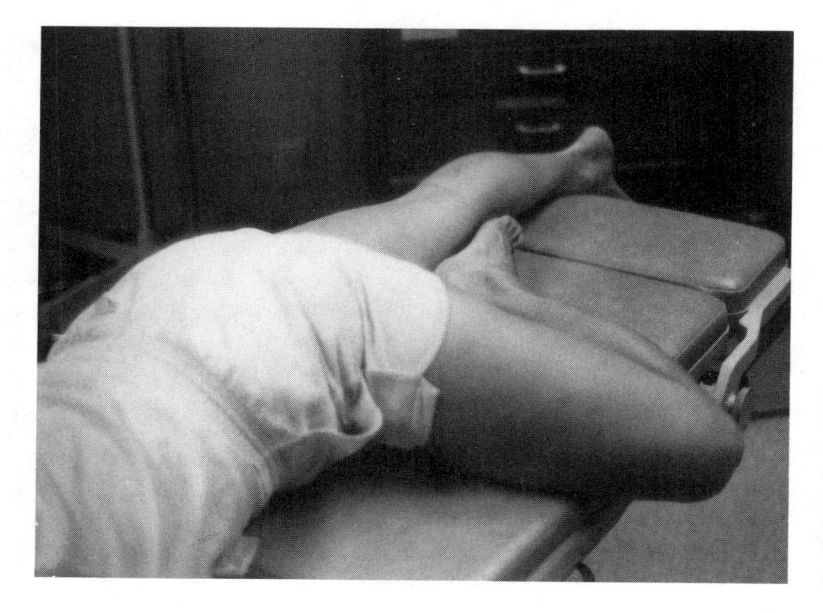

Figure 17.4.
Flexing the contralateral knee and hip will rotate the ipsilateral posterior calcaneal surface so that it is parallel with a frontal plane.

17-20
The total STJ ROM is measured so that the _____ _____ of that joint can be calculated.

neutral position

17-21
It is important, prior to making the calcaneal bisection, that the posterior aspect of the STJ be in the _____ plane.

frontal

17-22
This is accomplished by having the patient (*flex/extend*) their opposite _____ and _____.

flex, hip, knee

17-23
Once the patient is in the proper position, the bisection is made along the proximal two-thirds of the posterior calcaneal surface, while the STJ is maintained in its neutral position.

(The reason that the distal one-third is not used is that the fat pad surrounding that part of the calcaneus makes it nearly impossible to accurately define the posterior calcaneal borders in that area.)

17-24

The STJ neutral position is found by moving the foot by grasping the fifth metatarsal and:

A) observing the concave curves above and below the lateral malleolus (Fig. 17.5A). When the curves are of approximately equal concavity, the STJ is in its neutral position.

B) finding the point at which the STJ direction of motion changes (i.e., the plantarward motion of the calcaneus changes to a dorsalward motion) when going from a supinated to a pronated position (Fig. 17.5B). This has been likened to approaching a peak from one side, reaching it (the neutral position), and then going down the other side.

C) palpating the congruity of the talonavicular joint (TNJ) on its medial aspect. When the foot and STJ are supinated, the forefoot is adducted on the rearfoot, and there is an angular feel to the medial aspect of the TNJ. Conversely, when the foot and STJ are pronated, the forefoot becomes abducted on the rearfoot and an angularity is palpated that is the reverse of that observed with a supinated position. The neutral position is at the point of congruity where no angularity in either direction can be palpated.

Of the methods presented above for finding the STJ neutral position, A) and B) are the most reliable, and A) is the easier of the two.

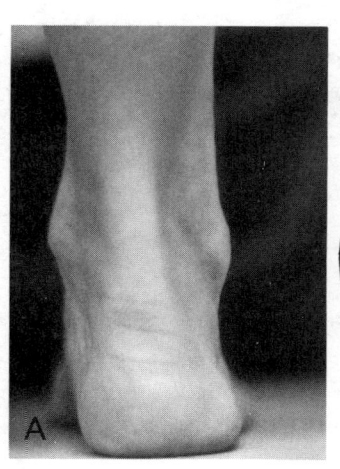

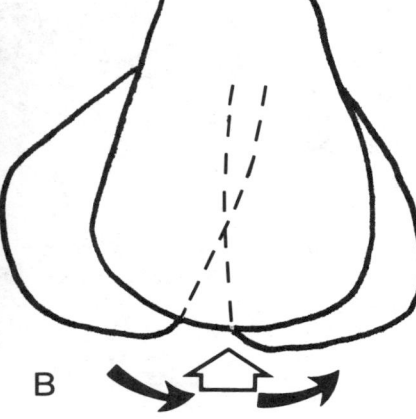

Figure 17.5.
A, Equal concavities above and below the lateral malleolus indicate a neutral STJ position. B, A reversal of the direction of calcaneal motion indicates a neutral STJ position.

17-25

The calcaneal bisection is made by palpating the medial and lateral borders of the (*proximal/distal*) two-thirds of the calcaneus (with the STJ neutral) and placing three dots to mark the bisection—one proximal, one distal, and one in between.

It is very important that the three dots be placed on the calcaneus while the examiner's eyes are directly above it (Fig. 17.6).

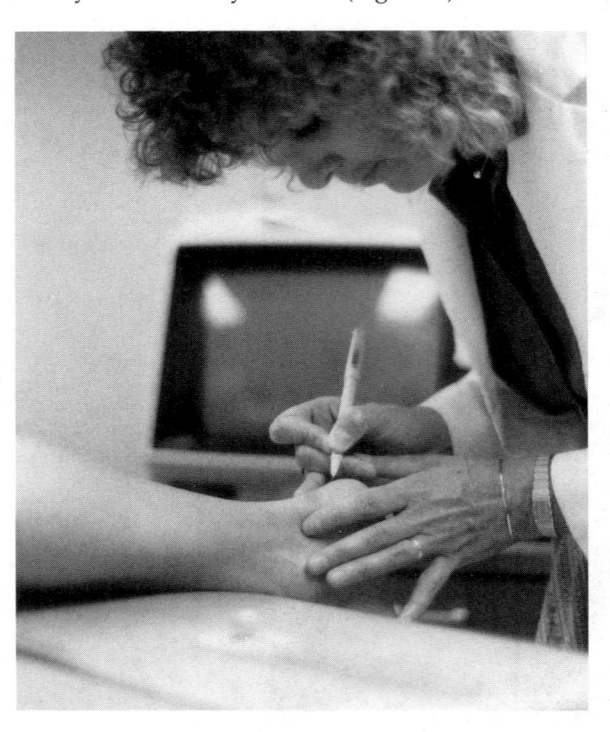

Figure 17.6.
To obtain a valid calcaneal bisection, the examiner's eyes must be directly above the calcaneus.

proximal

17-26

Each dot should be placed at the midpoint between the medial and lateral sides of the posterior aspect of the proximal _____ of the calcaneus.

two-thirds

17-27
After the dots have been placed properly (Fig. 17.7A), they should be rechecked to make certain that they are where they should be.

Then, connect the dots with a solid line and extend that line down the posterior one-third of the calcaneus (Fig. 17.7B). The line should appear straight and should be drawn without a straight edge. Paradoxically, use of a straight edge will distort the skin and usually result in a curved line.

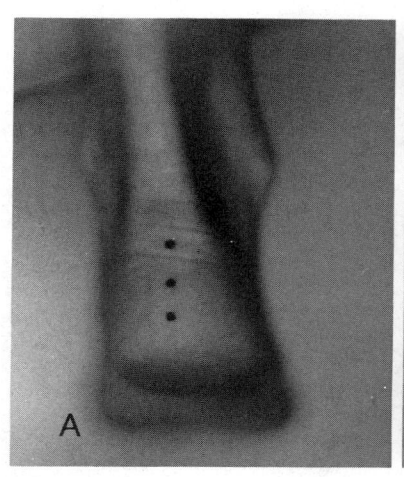

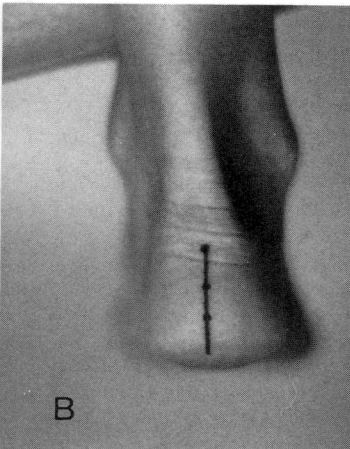

Figure 17.7.
A, Dots bisect the proximal two-thirds of the calcaneus. B, After connecting the bisecting dots, the line is extended down the distal posterior one-third of the calcaneus.

17-28
Next, the foot is grasped at the MTJ and is pronated and supinated, thus pronating and supinating the STJ.

It is important when performing this part of the exam that the foot be *dorsiflexed to resistance*, as the posterior part of the talar dome is narrower than the anterior portion and will allow artifactual frontal plane motion to be measured. By dorsiflexing the foot, the wider anterior part of the talar dome is locked into the ankle mortise. Thus, the only frontal plane motion measured is from the STJ.

17-29
In extending the line down the posterior one-third of the calcaneus, a straight edge (*should/should not*) be used.

should not

17-30
When pronating and supinating the foot to measure the STJ ROM, the foot should be grasped at the _____ joint.

midtarsal

17-31
In measuring the STJ ROM, it is important to maintain the foot _____ to resistance, so that there will be no artifactual frontal plane motion recorded.

dorsiflexed

17-32

The STJ is first placed in its maximally supinated position. The distal one-third of the bisection is the area that is looked at since it does not tend to move relative to the bone. The proximal two-thirds does move relative to the calcaneus with STJ motion. This causes the line to appear curved when the STJ is held in a position other than neutral (Fig. 17.8).

With the STJ maximally supinated, the distal one-third of the bisection is extended in a straight line up to the most proximal aspect of the calcaneus (Fig. 17.9A).

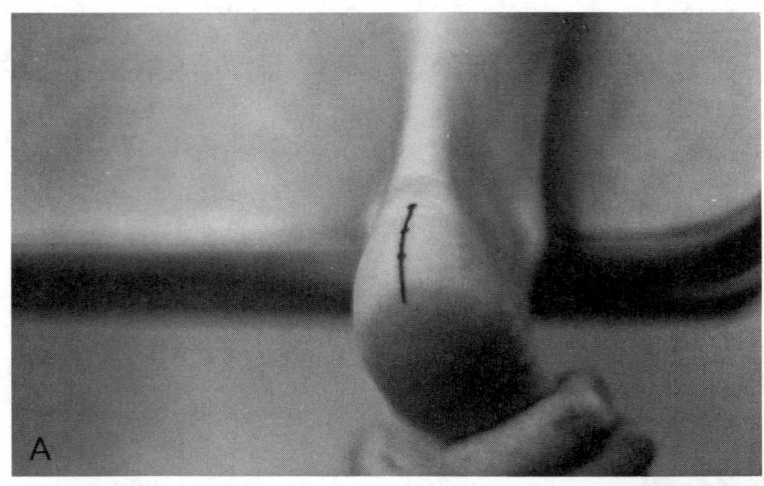

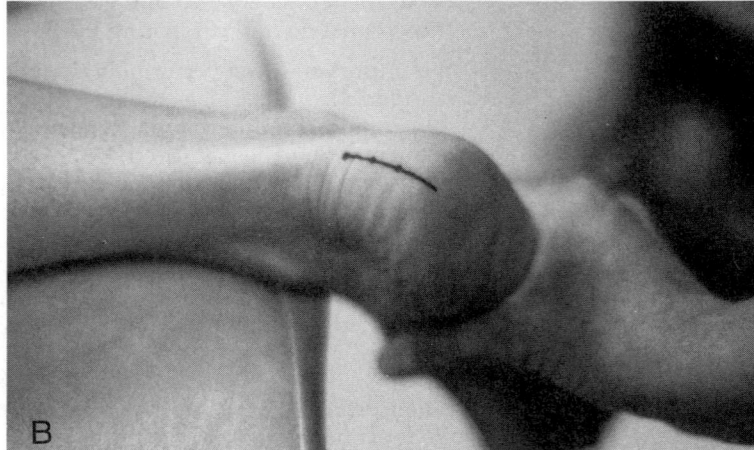

Figure 17.8.
A, With the STJ in a pronated position, the calcaneal line becomes curved. *B*, A supinated STJ position also causes curving of the calcaneal bisector.

17-33

The STJ is then placed in its maximally pronated position, and the distal one-third of the bisection is again extended up to the most proximal aspect of the calcaneus (Fig. 17.9B).

With the foot relaxed, these lines will appear as a "Y" with the original bisection in its middle.

The purpose of extending the lines proximally in this manner is to allow easier visualization of the calcaneal bisector in the maximally pronated and supinated positions.

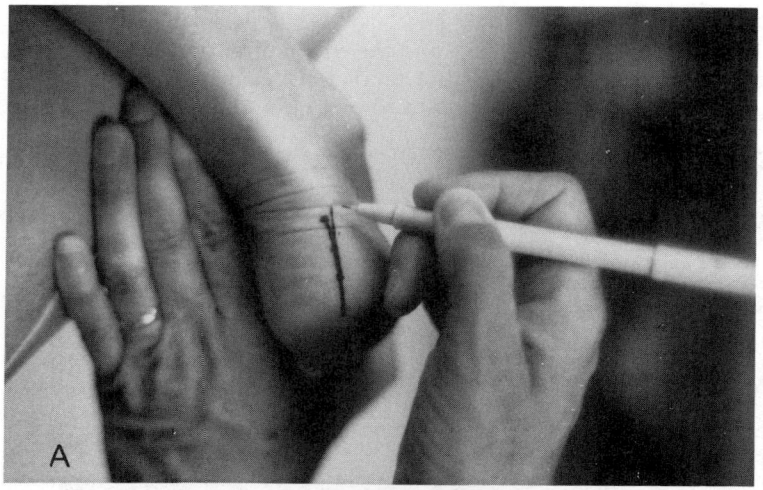

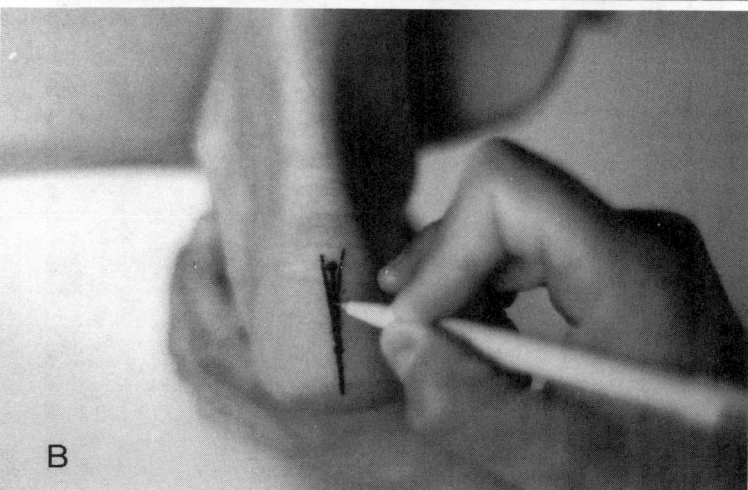

Figure 17.9.
A, Appearance of the bisections after the distal one-third is extended proximally with the STJ maximally supinated. B, Appearance of the bisections after the distal one-third is extended proximally with the STJ maximally pronated.

17-34

To measure the STJ total ROM, the foot is first dorsiflexed to resistance, the MTJ area is grasped, and the foot and STJ are supinated maximally. One arm of the goniometer (a.k.a. tractograph) is placed parallel with the straight calcaneal bisector. The other arm of the goniometer is placed parallel with the posterior leg bisector, and the resulting angle is measured (Fig. 17.10A). This is repeated with the STJ maximally pronated (Fig. 17.10B).

(The hinge of the goniometer is placed at the point where the bisectors of the posterior calcaneus and posterior distal one-third of the leg intersect).

The total ROM is calculated, and the STJ neutral position is defined as that point that divides the medial two-thirds of motion (i.e., _____) from the lateral one-third of motion (i.e., _____).

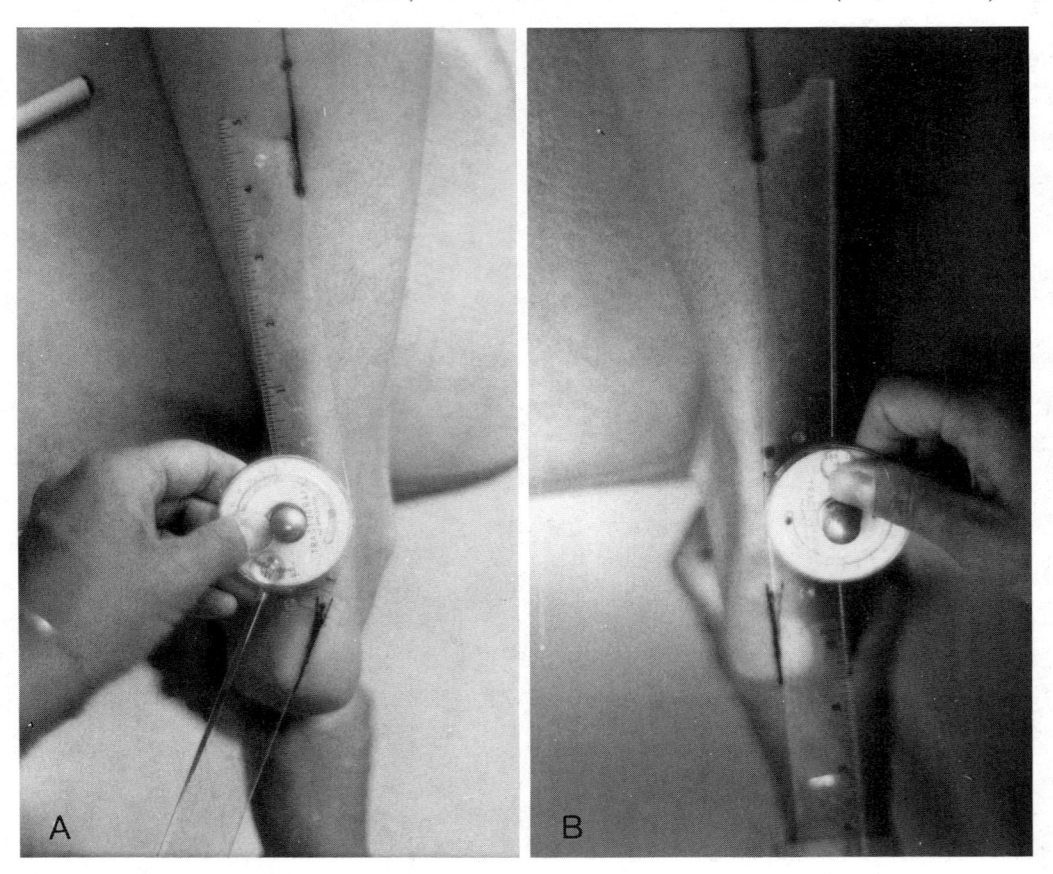

Figure 17.10. *A,* Calcaneal angulation from the leg bisection is measured with the STJ held maximally supinated. *B,* The STJ is then maximally pronated, and the calcaneal angulation from the leg is again measured.

supination, pronation

17-35
The minimum total STJ ROM necessary for normal ambulation is 10° (i.e., a range of 8°–12°) of motion.

Usually, the total STJ ROM (*is/is not*) symmetrical.

is

17-36
Another measurement that is taken is the *forefoot to rearfoot relationship*. This is an index of the _____ joint position.

midtarsal

17-37
In practice, this is usually done after the calcaneal bisection (with the STJ in its neutral position) is made. (There are fewer lines to confuse the eye.)

The foot is held by the fifth metatarsal and dorsiflexed to resistance. The forefoot is inverted to resistance (Fig. 17.11A) and then slowly everted until the STJ reaches its neutral position (Fig. 17.11B).

The reason that the foot must go from a supinated position in the direction of pronation is to keep the MTJ maximally pronated at both of its axes.

If the direction of motion was one of supination (i.e., starting at a maximally pronated position and going toward a more supinated position), there would be some inversion about the MTJ longitudinal axis, thus distorting the true forefoot to rearfoot relationship as we define it.

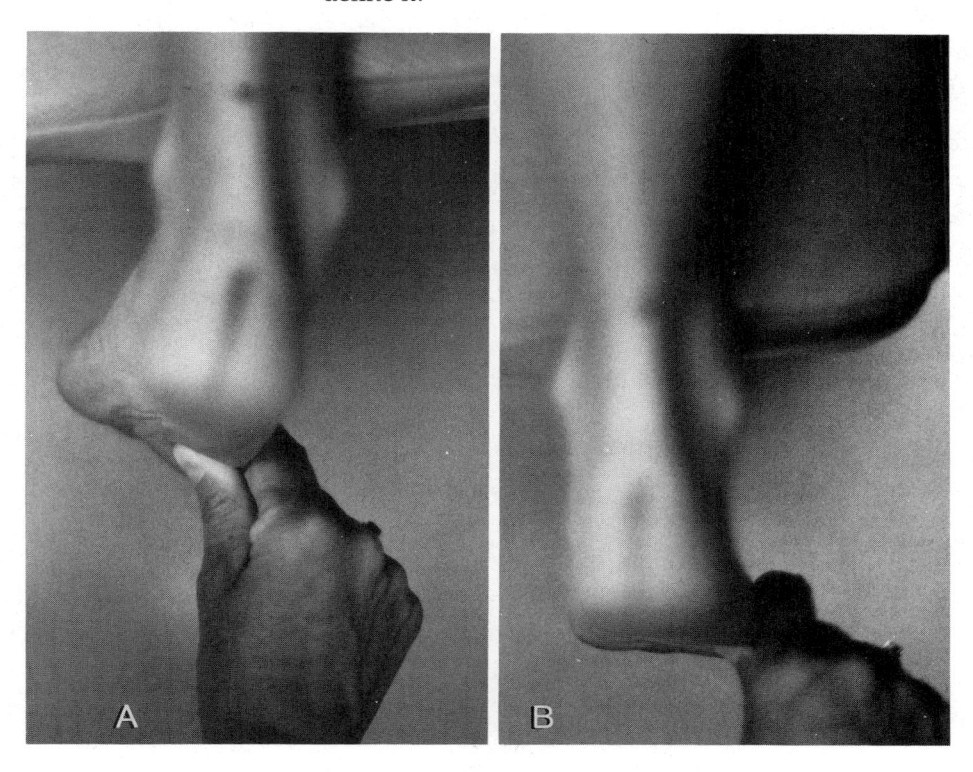

Figure 17.11. *A*, Forefoot inverted to resistance. *B*, Eversion is stopped when the STJ reaches its neutral position.

17-38

So, to measure the forefoot to rearfoot relationship and thus index the MTJ position, the fifth metatarsal is grasped, the foot is _____ to resistance and maximally _____.

dorsiflexed, supinated

17-39

The foot is then moved in the direction of _____ until the STJ reaches its _____ _____.

pronation, neutral position

17-40

At this point, the forefoot to rearfoot position is measured and recorded. The forefoot to rearfoot relationship is the angulation between the plantar plane of the rearfoot and the plantar plane of the forefoot.

The plantar plane of the rearfoot is a perpendicular to the calcaneal bisector. The plantar plane of the forefoot is the plane between metatarsal heads one and five if the first ray motion is normal and between metatarsal heads two and five if the first ray motion is abnormal.

17-41

Remember, when measuring the forefoot to rearfoot relationship, always make sure that the MTJ is maximally _____ at both of its axes.

pronated

17-42

The forefoot to rearfoot relationship is the angle between the _____ plane of the forefoot and the plantar plane of the _____.

17-43

plantar, rearfoot

The forefoot to rearfoot relationship (an index of _____ joint position) is measured with a goniometer or a forefoot measuring device.

If the goniometer is used, the arms are placed across the metatarsal heads with one parallel to the plantar plane of the forefoot and the other parallel to the plantar plane of the rearfoot (Fig. 17.12).

If the forefoot measuring device is used, the slit is placed over the calcaneal bisector, and the flat edge of the protractor is placed on the metatarsal heads.

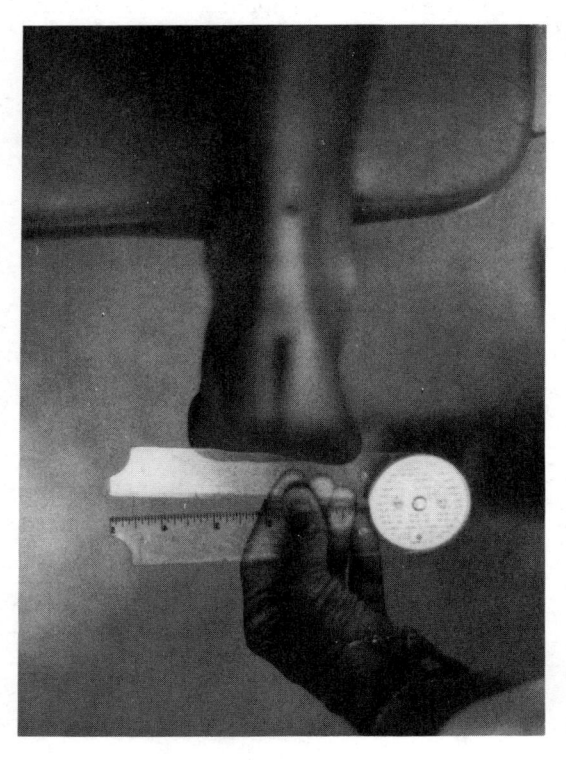

Figure 17.12. Measurement of the forefoot to rearfoot relationship.

17-44

midtarsal

In utilizing either device for this measurement, it is imperative to keep the foot _____ to resistance and the MTJ maximally _____ about both of its axes.

17-45

dorsiflexed, pronated

Prior to taking the forefoot to rearfoot measurement, it is generally a good idea to estimate the relationship and then correlate this with the measured findings. This helps prevent measurements with unintended MTJ supination from occurring.

17-46

If the plantar plane of the forefoot is inverted relative to the plantar plane of the rearfoot with the STJ in its neutral position and the MTJ maximally pronated about both of its axes, this is called a forefoot _____ deformity.

varus

17-47
A forefoot valgus deformity is defined as the plantar plane of the forefoot being _____ relative to the plantar plane of the rearfoot with the STJ in its neutral position and the MTJ maximally pronated about both of its axes.

everted

17-48
Another parameter which needs to be evaluated in the NWB biomechanical examination is the *first ray ROM*.

Normally, there should be equal amounts of dorsiflexion (coupled with _____) and plantarflexion (coupled with _____).

17: BIOMECHANICAL EXAMINATION: NON-WEIGHTBEARING ASSESSMENT 229

inversion, eversion

17-49

First ray ROM is measured by first dorsiflexing the foot to resistance and then bringing the STJ into its neutral position (as was done in the forefoot to rearfoot evaluation).

While maintaining the foot in this position, the second through fifth metatarsal heads are stabilized with one hand. (Fig. 17.13*A*). The other hand grasps the first metatarsal head and moves it in dorsal and plantar directions to resistance (Fig. 17.13*B* and Fig. 17.13*C*).

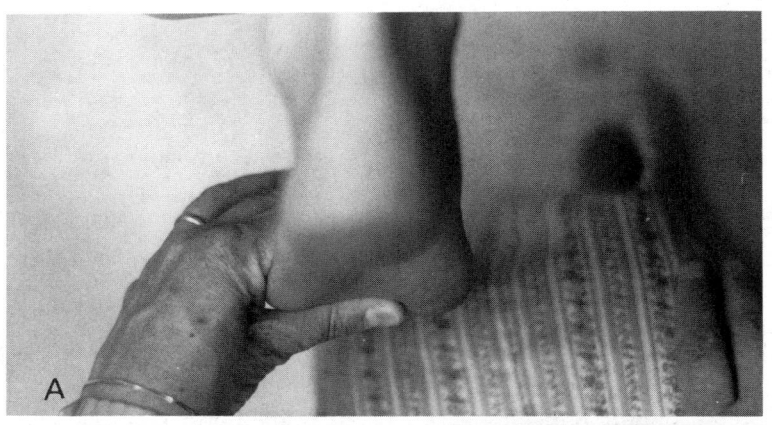

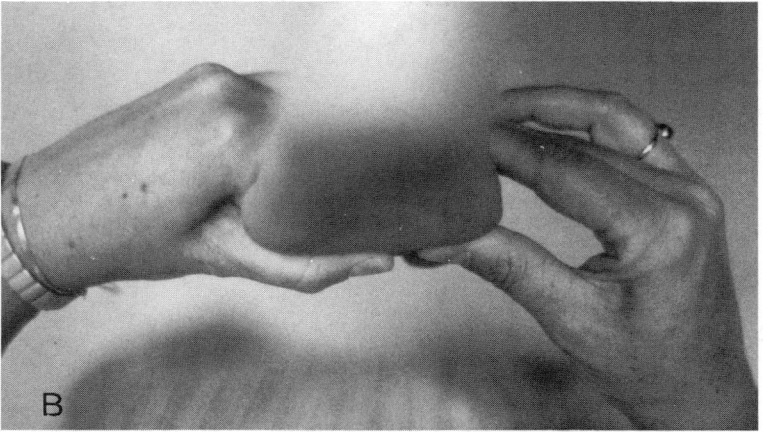

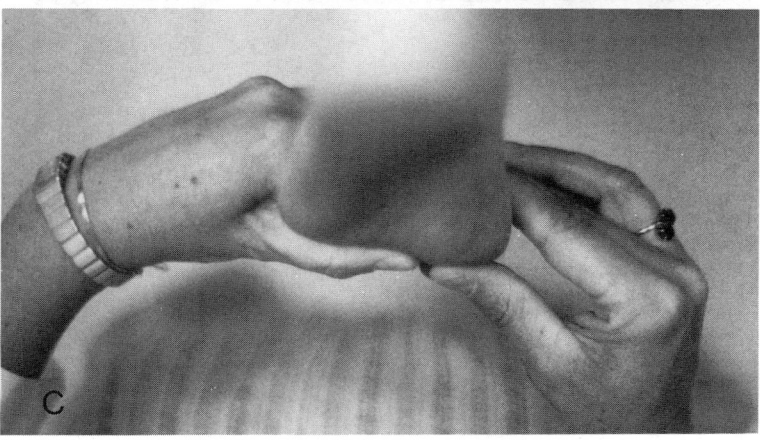

Figure 17.13.
A, The lesser metatarsal heads are stabilized with the foot dorsiflexed to resistance and the STJ in its neutral position. *B*, The first metatarsal head is moved dorsally to resistance. *C*, The first metatarsal head is then moved plantarly to resistance.

17-50
In examining the first ray ROM, the STJ is maintained in its _____ _____, and the foot is dorsiflexed to resistance.

neutral position

17-51
The _____ through the _____ metatarsal heads are stabilized with one hand while the other hand grasps the _____ metatarsal head.

second, fifth, first

17-52
The first metatarsal head is then moved in _____ and _____ directions until resistance is felt in each direction.

dorsal, plantar

17-53
The three things noted while performing this examination are:

A) the level of the first metatarsal head relative to the second metatarsal head in the starting (or neutral) position. Normally, these two metatarsal heads will be even with each other. Using the thumbnails as an index of metatarsal head position is a standard practice in the evaluation of first ray ROM.

B) the amount of dorsal excursion. Normally, this will be about 5 mm.

C) the amount of plantar excursion. This will normally be equal to the dorsal excursion—i.e., about _____ mm.

5

17-54
If there was more dorsiflexion of the first ray than plantarflexion (Fig. 17.14), this would be called a _____ _____ _____ deformity.

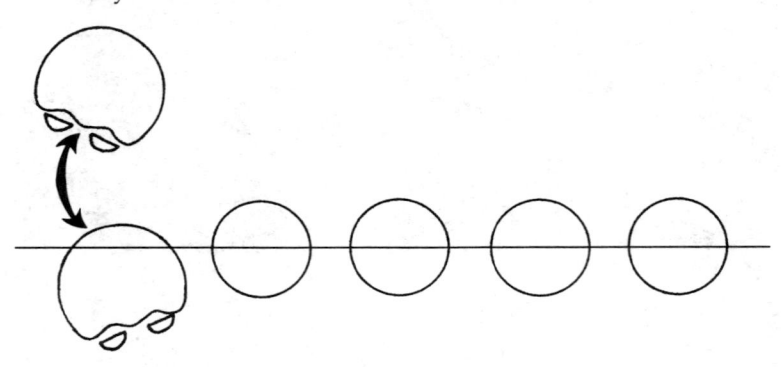

Figure 17.14.

metatarsus primus elevatus	**17-55** If there was more plantarflexion observed than there was dorsiflexion of the first ray (Fig. 17.15), this would be called a _____ _____ deformity.

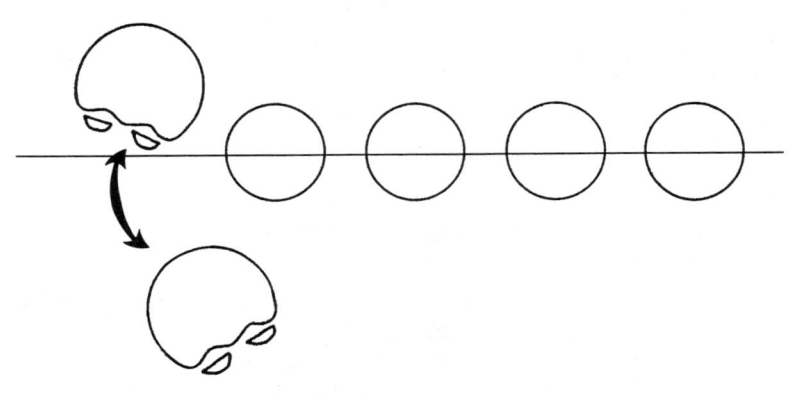

Figure 17.15.

plantarflexed first ray	**17-56** The normal total ROM of the first ray is usually about _____ mm.
10	**17-57** The first ray usually has _____ mm of dorsiflexion and _____ mm of plantarflexion available.
5, 5	**17-58** Remember when measuring the forefoot to rearfoot relationship, if there is an abnormal first ray ROM, the plantar plane of the forefoot must be considered as the plane between the _____ and fifth metatarsal heads.
second	**17-59** A final measurement needed in the NWB biomechanical examination is that of *malleolar torsion*. Malleolar torsion is a measurement which is an index to the amount of tibial torsion (i.e., growth in the transverse plane) which has occurred.
	17-60 Malleolar torsion is an index of tibial growth in the _____ plane.
transverse	**17-61** The actual tibial torsion cannot be directly measured, so instead we measure the _____ _____.
malleolar torsion	**17-62** In the adult, malleolar torsion is normally 13° to 18° externally rotated. This is called external malleolar torsion.

17-63

Malleolar torsion is measured with the patient in the supine position. The patient's knee must be parallel with a frontal plane—i.e., the posterior aspects of the femoral condyles should rest equally on the examination table.

The malleolar torsion is measured with either a goniometer or a gravity goniometer.

Normal malleolar torsion is in the range of _____° to _____° _____ rotated.

13, 18, externally

17-64

Recall that the tibia and talus move together in normal closed kinetic chain (CKC) STJ function.

If, for example, the position of the tibia is *relatively* internally rotated (e.g., 8° of external rotation), the amount of STJ pronation available in closed kinetic chain function will be severely limited. This would be due to the talus being pulled by the tibia into the position that it would assume with maximal pronation. Since the talus is already there, further pronation is impossible. When there is a relatively internally rotated malleolar position, it is called simply lack of malleolar torsion.

The converse would be true with regard to excessive external malleolar torsion and its effect in limiting CKC STJ supination.

17-65

In measuring the amount of malleolar torsion, the medial and lateral malleoli must be bisected (Fig. 17.16A and Fig. 17.16B).

If the standard goniometer is to be used, the bisections must be extended distally, taking care to keep them parallel with the supporting surface. With the standard goniometer held at the plantar aspect of the patient's foot, one arm of the goniometer is held so as to connect the two malleolar bisections and the other arm is held parallel with the surface of the examining table (and therefore with the posterior aspects of the femoral condyles) (Fig. 17.16C). The angle is then read.

If a gravity goniometer is used, the tips of the calipers are placed on the bisections of the malleoli, and the angle is then read at the tip of the hanging needle.

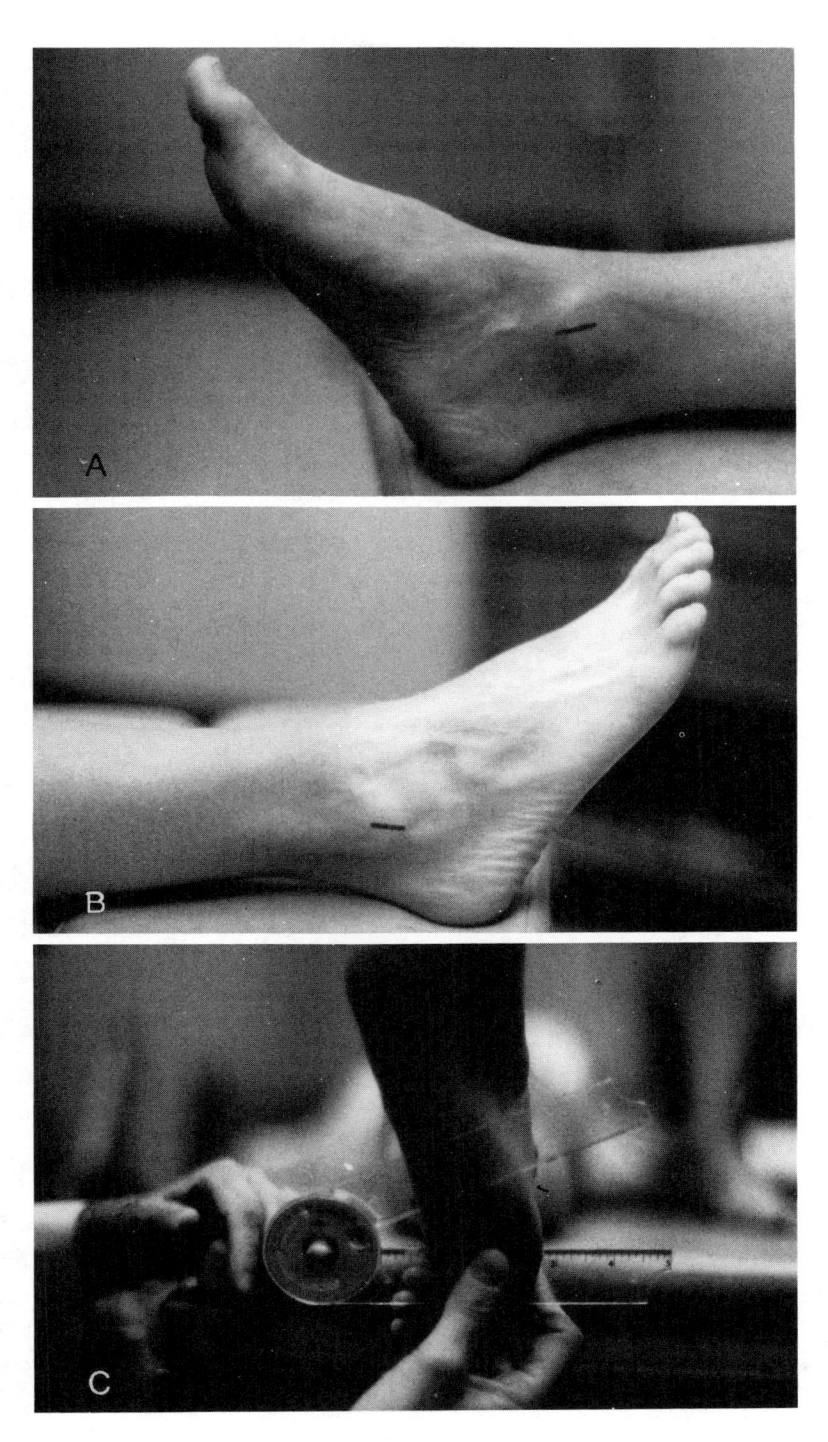

Figure 17.16.
A, Bisection of the medial malleolus. *B,* Bisection of the lateral malleolus. *C,* Measurement of malleolar torsion.

second

17-66
If there is a lack of malleolar torsion (i.e., a relatively *externally/internally* rotated malleolar position), there is usually an accompanying limitation in CKC STJ _____.

internally, pronation

17-67
This concludes the chapter.

In the next chapter, the weightbearing part of the biomechanical examination will be presented.

Questions

FRAME 17-2

1. In most patients, foot joint ROM is asymmetrical.
   a. true
   b. false

FRAME 17-4

2. The criteria for normalcy are not often found clinically.
   a. true
   b. false

FRAME 17-6

3. The minimum amount of ankle joint dorsiflexion with the knee extended necessary for normal ambulation to occur is:
   a. 0°
   b. 5°
   c. 10°
   d. 15°
   e. 20°

FRAMES 17-9—17-11

4. If the amount of ankle joint dorsiflexion is the same with the knee flexed and extended, the most likely diagnosis is:
   a. gastocnemius equinus
   b. ankle equinus
   c. soleus equinus
   d. a and b
   e. b and c

FRAMES 17-11 AND 17-12

5. A gastrocnemius equinus will cause:
   a. more ankle dorsiflexion with the knee extended
   b. more ankle dorsiflexion with the knee flexed
   c. equal amounts of ankle dorsiflexion with the knee flexed and extended
   d. more ankle plantarflexion with the knee extended
   e. more ankle plantarflexion with the knee flexed

FRAME 17-32

6. The distal one-third of the calcaneal bisection does not tend to move relative to the calcaneus with STJ motion.
   a. true
   b. false

FRAME 17-35

7. The minimum total STJ ROM necessary for normal ambulation is:
   a. 0°
   b. 5°
   c. 10°
   d. 15°
   e. 20°

FRAME 17-37

8. In assessing the forefoot to rearfoot relationship, it is necessary that the foot be moved from a pronated to a supinated position before being measured.
   a. true
   b. false

FRAME 17-59

9. Malleolar torsion is an index of:
   a. MTJ position
   b. STJ position
   c. fibular torsion
   d. tibial torsion
   e. femoral torsion

FRAME 17-62

10. Which of the following represents an abnormal internal malleolar torsion?
    a. 11°
    b. 13°
    c. 15°
    d. a and b
    e. b and c

Answers

1. b
2. a
3. c
4. e
5. b
6. a
7. c
8. b
9. d
10. a

CHAPTER 18

Biomechanical Examination: Weightbearing Assessment

- angle and base of gait—definition and determination
- neutral calcaneal stance position—definition and measurement
- relaxed calcaneal stance position—definition and measurement
- tibial varum—definition and measurement
- gait evaluation
- identification of apropulsive gait

18-1
There are four parameters which must be assessed in the weight-bearing (WB) biomechanical assessment:

A) Neutral Calcaneal Stance Position (NCSP)
B) Relaxed Calcaneal Stance Position (RCSP)
C) Tibial Curvature (Varum or Valgum)
D) Gait

18-2
The NCSP, RCSP, and tibial varum are measured in the patient's *angle and base of gait*.

18-3
The angle and base of gait are necessary to measure the _____ _____ stance position, _____ _____ stance position, and the amount (if any) of tibial varum.

neutral calcaneal, relaxed calcaneal

18-4
The patient's angle and base of gait are best determined by observing them in gait over a period of a minute or two.

The angle of gait is the number of degrees that the foot is deviated from the line of progression of gait.

Normally, the foot is *between 7° and 10° abducted from the line of progression*.

18-5

The base of gait is defined as the space between the malleoli during the midstance period. This is usually about *one and one-half inches*.

The angle of gait is usually between _____ and _____ degrees (*adducted/abducted*).

7, 10 abducted

18-6

By taking the WB measurements in the angle and base of gait, we are duplicating the position in which the foot must function during gait. The angle and base of gait also allow *standardization* (and, therefore, *reproducibility* of values in the WB biomechanical assessment) between different physicians.

(Incidentally, for the same reason of insuring reproducibility of biomechanical values, foot radiographs are taken with the patient in the angle and base of gait.)

18-7

The patient is observed and the angle and base of gait are recorded. The patient is then placed on a platform so that the clinician's eyes may be level with the patient's calcanei (Fig. 18.1). The patient is then placed in the angle and base of gait recorded earlier.

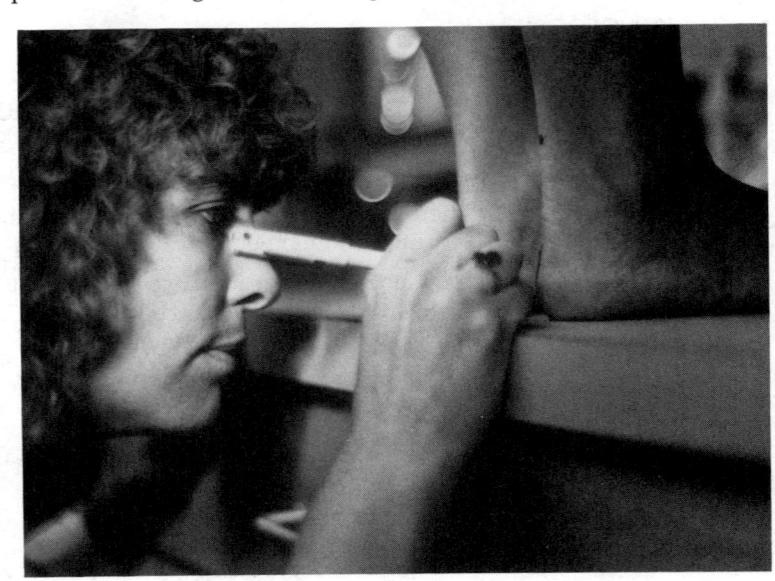

Figure 18.1.
For a valid weight-bearing assessment, the examiner's eyes must be level with the patient's calcanei.

18-8

In order to perform the WB biomechanical measurements involving the calcaneus, it is necessary to rebisect the calcaneus. The non-weightbearing bisections are usually distorted enough by weightbearing so as to be inaccurate.

In rebisecting the calcaneus, the same method should be used as was described in Chapter 17. The (*proximal/distal*) (*one-third/two-thirds*) should be bisected by placing three dots over the posterior surface initially, then connecting the dots and extending the bisection distally.

(Remember, all WB biomechanical measurements must be taken with the patient in his or her angle and base of gait.)

18-9

(Fig. 18.2. See preceding frame.)

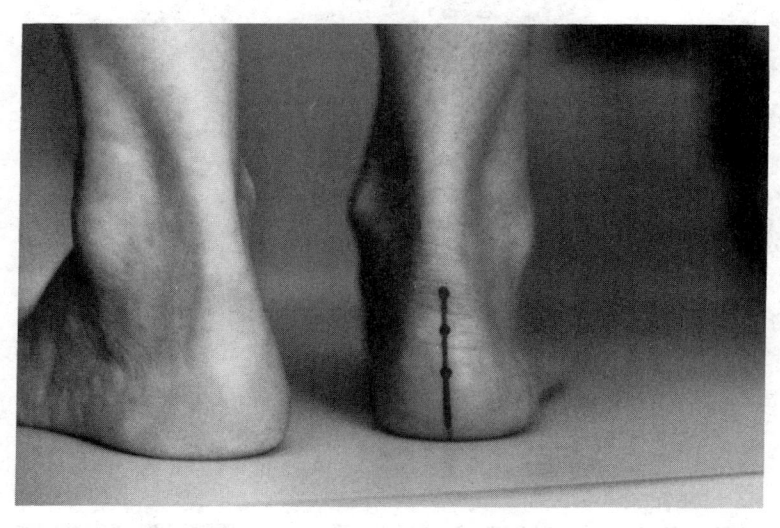

Figure 18.2.
The proximal two-thirds of the calcaneus is bisected at three points. The points are then connected, and the line is extended distally.

proximal, two-thirds

The *neutral calcaneal stance position (NCSP)* is defined as the angular relationship between the calcaneus and the ground with STJ in its neutral position and the patient standing in the angle and base of gait.

To find the NCSP, the calcaneus should be rebisected with the STJ in its neutral position with the patient standing.

The easiest way to place the STJ in its neutral position is to have the patient slowly roll the foot in and out while the examiner observes the concavities above and below the lateral malleolus (Fig. 18.3). When these concavities are equal, the STJ is in its neutral position, and the patient should be instructed to hold that position while the same procedure is repeated on the opposite foot.

A way of double-checking the NCSP is to look at the lateral aspect of the forefoot relative to the lateral aspect of the rearfoot. The forefoot should be neither abducted or adducted on the rearfoot as it would be respectively with STJ pronation or supination.

After achieving the NCSP in both feet, the concavities above and below the _____ _____ should again be checked to confirm that the patient has not inadvertently changed position in the interim.

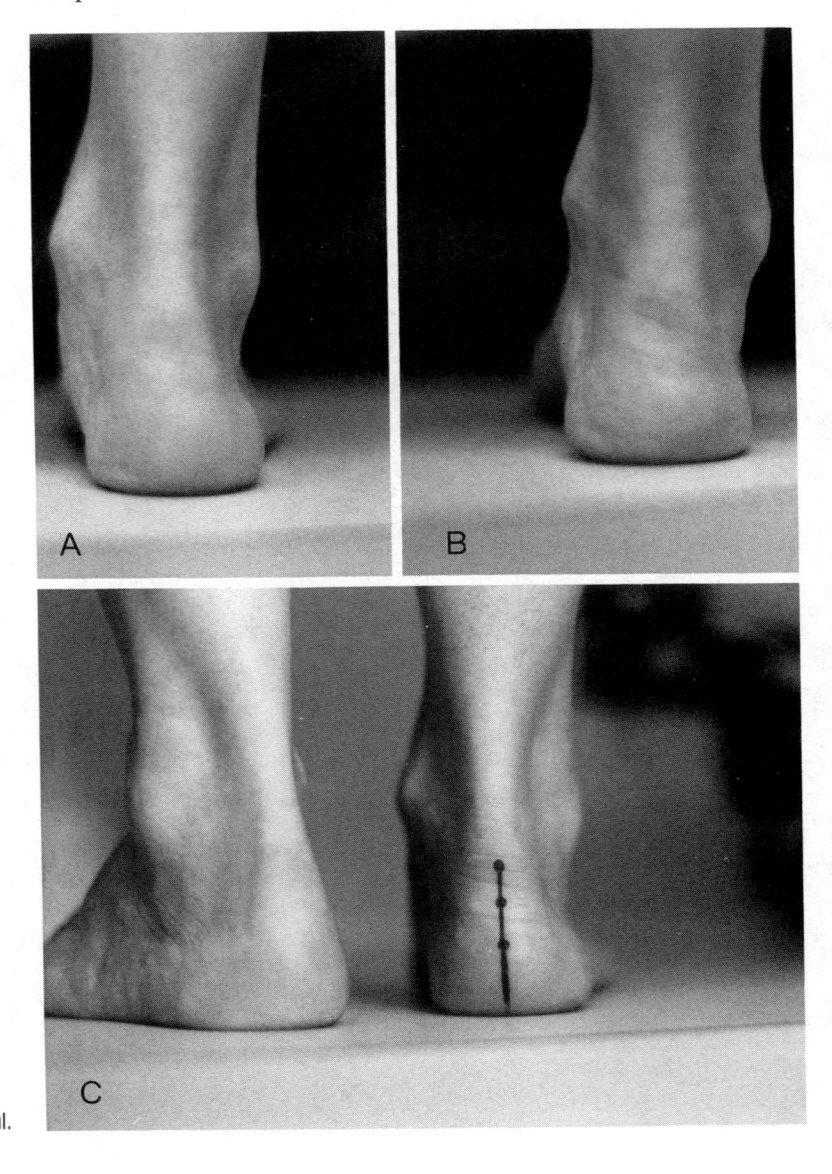

Figure 18.3.
A, In a pronated position, the concavity inferior to the lateral malleolus is more everted than the one superior. *B,* In a supinated position, the inferior concavity is more inverted than is the superior. *C,* When the STJ is in its neutral position, the inferior and superior concavities appear equal.

18: BIOMECHANICAL EXAMINATION: WEIGHTBEARING ASSESSMENT 241

lateral malleoli

18-10
In bisecting the calcaneus with the patient standing, it is very important to have the examiner's eyes in the same plane as the posterior surface of the calcaneus. In the NWB exam, it was possible to achieve this by having the patient flex the opposite _____ and _____.

hip, knee

18-11
With the patient standing, the examiner must move in order to place his or her eyes parallel with the posterior surface of the calcaneus.

(When the patient stands in the angle of gait, the posterior surface of the calcaneus will be rotated further away from a frontal plane than if the patient stood with the feet parallel to a sagittal plane.)

18-12
The angular relationship between the calcaneus and the (perpendicular to the) ground—with the patient standing relaxed in the angle and base of gait—is called the _____ _____ _____ _____.

relaxed calcaneal stance position

18-13
The NCSP is measured with the patient standing in the angle and base of gait with the STJ in its _____ position.

neutral

18-14
The NCSP is measured by placing one arm of the goniometer parallel with the supporting surface and the other arm parallel with the calcaneal bisection (Fig. 18.4).

Alternate methods of measuring the NCSP position include the use of a gravity goniometer or a protractor. All methods measure the angulation between the calcaneal bisection and a perpendicular to the supporting surface.

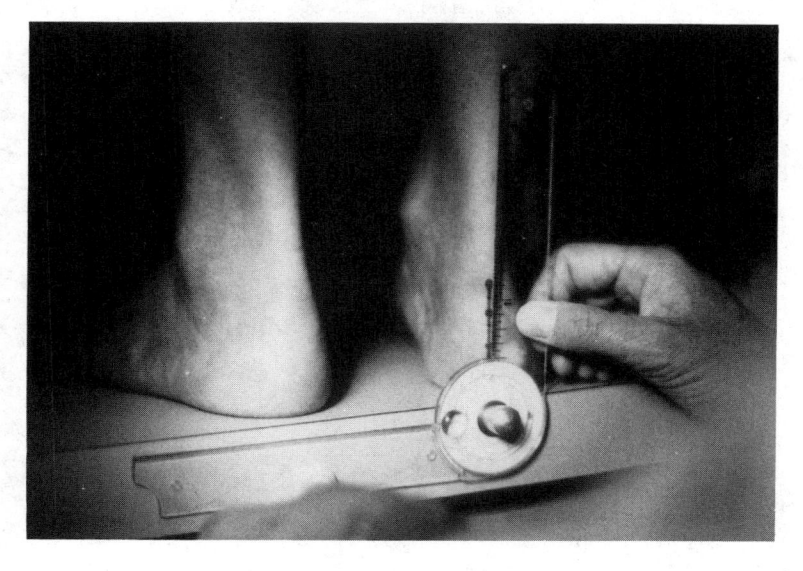

Figure 18.4.
Measuring the NCSP.

18-15
The RCSP is measured with the patient standing in the _____ and _____ of gait with the STJ in a _____ position.

angle, base, relaxed

18-16
The RCSP is most easily accomplished after measuring the NCSP by instructing the patient to remain where they are standing but to relax the feet and ankles.

18-17
The RCSP is measured in the same manner as is the NCSP (Fig. 18.5).

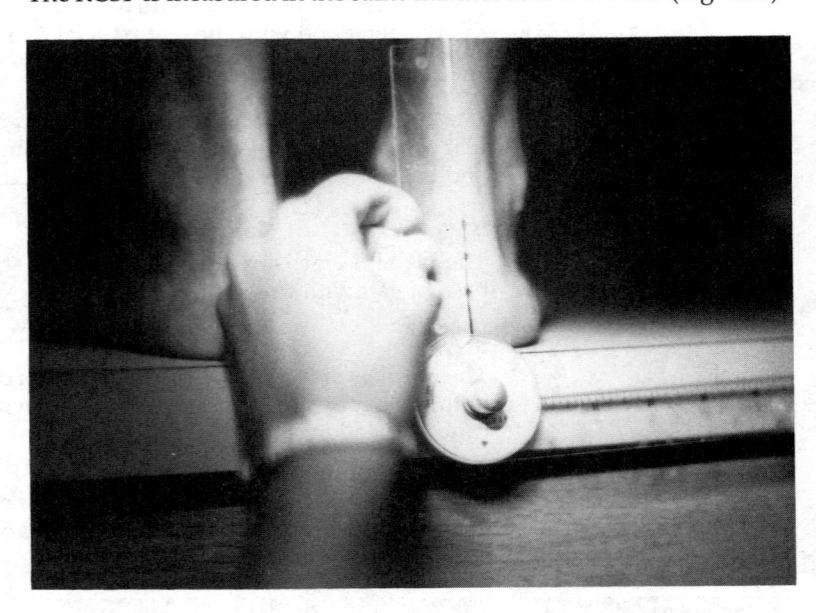

Figure 18.5. Measuring the RCSP.

18-18
The last measurement that is needed in the static WB biomechanical evaluation is that of *tibial varum*. (Tibial valgum is relatively rare and will not be addressed here, although the method of measuring it is the same as for tibial varum.)

18-19
Tibial varum is defined as an abnormal _____ plane orientation of the tibia due to bowing in that plane.

The distal aspect of the tibia is (*inverted/everted*) relative to the proximal aspect of the tibia.

frontal, inverted

18-20
Tibial varum is measured with the patient in the angle and base of gait with the foot maintained in the NCSP.

For this measurement, the posterior aspect of the leg must be bisected. To bisect the posterior aspect of the leg (i.e., the tibia), the examiner must be directly posterior to the patient's leg.

18-21

The knee is bisected on its posterior aspect.

Next, the ankle is bisected on its posterior aspect at the malleolar level.

A dot is then placed on an imaginary line which connects the points on the ankle and the knee. (This is simply to make the assessment easier and perhaps more accurate.)

One arm of the goniometer is placed on the imaginary line between the ankle bisection and the dot above, and the other arm is placed perpendicular to the supporting surface.

Alternately, the base of the gravity goniometer is placed on the imaginary line between the dot at the ankle and the dot above. The angle is then read at the tip of the hanging needle.

18-22

Remember, when measuring tibial varum, the examiner should place the patient in the _____ calcaneal stance position and the angle and base of gait.

neutral

18-23

Remember to correlate the findings of the static WB examination with the other portions of the biomechanical examination.

Generally, there (*should/should not*) be relative symmetry between the findings on both sides.

should

18-24

To learn the gait evaluation adequately, it is especially important to observe many patients with an experienced clinician. This given, the elements of the gait evaluation will be mentioned, along with some of the more important abnormal findings that may be presented in the course of this examination.

It is important in this examination, as in most others, to have a *systematic manner of observation*.

18-25

In order to adequately perform a gait evaluation, it is optimal to have about 50 feet of well-polished floor surface for the patient to walk on. Overhead lighting is the best to use for this examination.

Since many patients will unconsciously try to please the physician by "walking right," it is a good idea to have the patient walk up and down the examination area for a few minutes. This gives them a chance to fatigue slightly which better reflects the normal state in which they ambulate.

Remember, it is important to have a _____ manner (or approach) in the gait evaluation.

systematic

18-26
One easy way of maintaining a systematic approach in the gait evaluation is to start observations at the head and work down to the feet.

In observing the head, note whether or not there is any *head tilt*. If there is, it may reflect scoliosis, neurologic deficit involving the extraocular muscles, degenerative joint disease, neuromuscular disease, etc.

The point here is that the head should be held straight in the midline, with no tilt toward either side (Fig. 18.6).

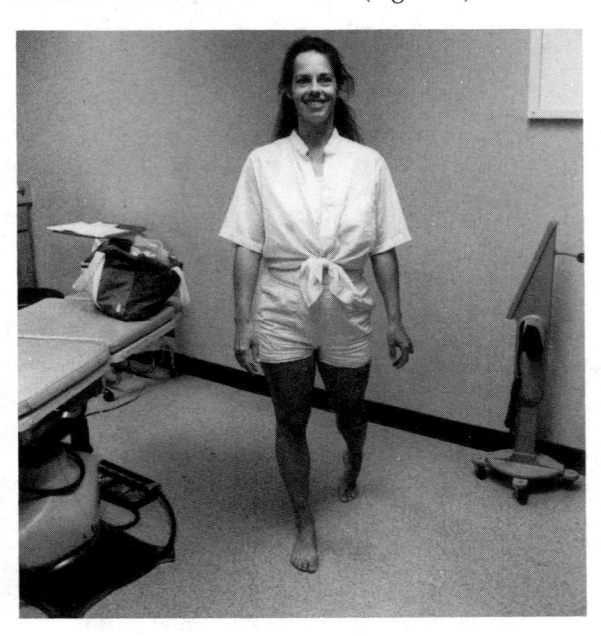

Figure 18.6.
The patient's head and shoulders should be held straight and level respectively.

18-27
The patient's *shoulders should be held level with one another* (Fig. 18.6). (An inequality in the shoulder level may point most prominently toward a scoliotic process or a functional or structural limb length discrepancy.)

18-28
Normally, the head should be held _____ in the midline, and the shoulders should be _____ with each other.

straight, level

18-29
The pelvis and trunk should be observed for *symmetrical rotation*. (Asymmetrical rotation may indicate a variance in the normal weight transfer sequence, such as that seen with abnormal propulsive STJ pronation.)

Additionally, the *iliac crests should be on an equal level with one another*. (Limb length discrepancy is one entity that will cause the iliac crest level to be unequal.)

18: BIOMECHANICAL EXAMINATION: WEIGHTBEARING ASSESSMENT

18-30
The knee should remain primarily in the sagittal plane during the gait cycle.

(If the femur is internally rotated, the knee will remain in an internally rotated position. If the medial hamstrings are tight, the knee will deviate internally just prior to heel contact.)

18-31
To briefly review, during the gait cycle, the iliac crest height is usually (*equal/unequal*).

equal

18-32
The pelvis and trunk normally exhibit (*symmetrical/assymetrical*) rotation during gait.

symmetrical

18-33
The knee normally functions in the _____ plane during gait.

sagittal

18-34
Sudden internal rotation of the knee just prior to heel contact may indicate tight _____ _____.

medial hamstrings

18-35
The knee should be in a vertical plane which connects the longitudinal axis of the thigh and the longitudinal axis of the leg.

18-36
If the knees are bowed in on a frontal plane (i.e., "knock-knees") and the legs are abducted relative to the thighs, this is called a *genu valgum* deformity (Fig. 18.7).

(Genu valgum may be associated with coxa vara—a more horizontal attitude of the femoral head and neck.)

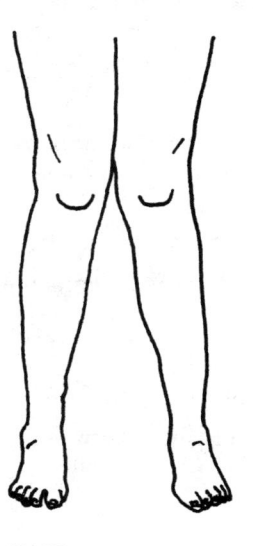

Figure 18.7.
Genu valgum.

18-37
"Knock-knees" or genu _____ defines the condition in which the knees are bowed (*in/out*) on a _____ plane.

valgum, in, frontal

18-38
The converse of genu valgum is *genu varum*.

Genu varum refers to a condition in which the knees are bowed out on a frontal plane (Fig. 18.8).

(Genu varum may be associated with coxa valga—a more vertical orientation of the femoral head and neck.)

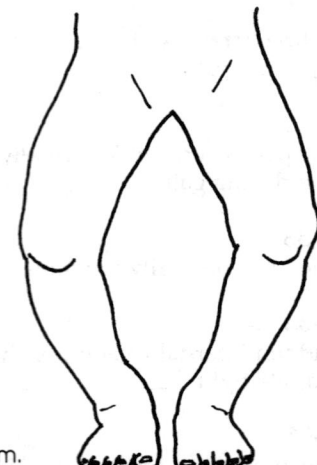

Figure 18.8.
Genu varum.

18-39
Hyperextension of the knee is called *genu recurvatum* and may be observed in gait as well as during the static portion of the WB biomechanical assessment.

(In genu recurvatum, the concavity faces anteriorly.)

18-40
Deformities of the knee—such as bowing outward on a frontal plane (i.e., genu _____) or hyperextension of the knee (i.e., genu _____)—will affect tibial position and motion.

varum, recurvatum

18-41
Since the tibial and talar positions are closely related, anything which changes the normal vertical orientation of the tibia will affect the STJ via the talus.

The abnormal STJ function will then be reflected in the entire foot.

Remember, correlate all of the different portions of the biomechanical examination.

18-42
The angle and base of gait should be observed.

Normally, the angle of gait is between _____° and _____° abducted from the line of progression.

18-43

7, 10

The normal base of gait is usually around _____ inches.

(An excessively wide base of gait may be associated with states of diminished proprioceptive or vestibular function, among others.)

18-44

1½

The position and motion of the STJ should be carefully observed during the contact, midstance, and propulsive periods of the stance phase of gait.

Motion of the _____ in the frontal plane is used as an index of STJ motion.

18-45

calcaneus

At the beginning of the contact period, the calcaneus should be slightly (*inverted/everted*), thus indicating a slightly _____ STJ position.

18-46

inverted, supinated

During the contact period, the STJ should be (*pronating/supinating*).

18-47

(Fig. 18.9. See preceding frame.)

pronating

The STJ normally (*pronates/supinates*) during the midstance and propulsive periods of gait.

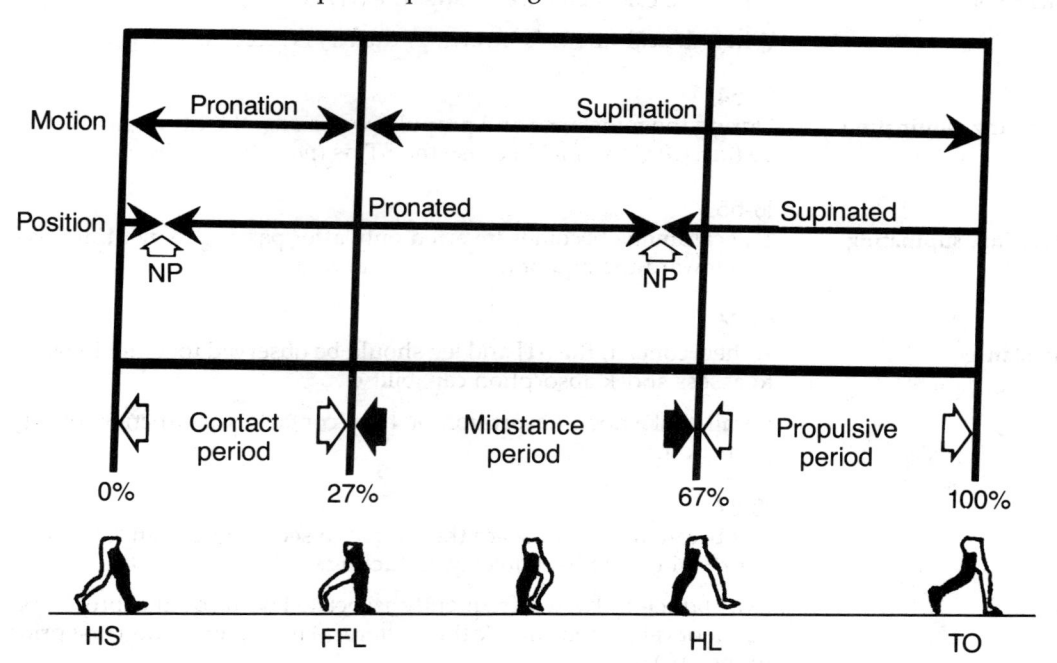

Figure 18.9. STJ motion and position during the stance phase of the gait cycle.

18-48
Thus, the most calcaneal eversion (i.e., STJ pronation) will occur toward the end of the contact period.

The STJ reaches its neutral position just before the (*beginning/end*) of the midstance period.

supinates

18-49
Before reaching its neutral position toward the end of the midstance period, the STJ is still in a (*pronated/supinated*) position.

end

18-50
After passing through its neutral position late in the midstance period, the STJ enters a supinated position which is reflected by the calcaneus being in an (*inverted/everted*) position.

pronated

18-51
During the propulsive period (after the STJ has passed its neutral position), the STJ continues (*pronating/supinating*) until just before toe off.

inverted

18-52
The index to STJ motion is the frontal plane motion of the _____.

supinating

18-53
When the calcaneus is everting, the STJ is _____.

When the calcaneus is inverting, the STJ is _____.

calcaneus

18-54
During the midstance and propulsive periods, the calcaneus should be (*inverting/everting*) because the STJ is (*pronating/supinating*).

pronating, supinating

18-55
The calcaneus becomes inverted only after passing its neutral position toward the end of the _____ period.

inverting, supinating

18-56
At heel contact, the STJ and leg should be observed together in order to assess shock absorption capability.

Recall that shock absorption at heel contact is a function of STJ pronation.

midstance

18-57
Just before toe off, observe the patient to see if there is an "*abductory twist*"—i.e., the heel quickly abducting.

(An abductory twist is frequently associated with equinus problems. Forefoot valgus may mimic this if there is sudden pronation just prior to toe off.)

18-58

The MTJ should be observed.

The lateral border of the forefoot will appear abducted on the rearfoot if the MTJ is in a pronated position.

Conversely, if the MTJ is in a supinated position, the lateral aspect of the forefoot will appear abducted on the rearfoot, thus giving a C-shaped appearance to the lateral aspect of the foot.

18-59

The MTJ should also be observed for sagittal plane subluxation.

This occurs with abnormal STJ pronation at the end of the midstance period and during the propulsive period.

The rearfoot is seen flexing over the forefoot since the stability of the foot as a rigid lever has been lost.

18-60

A C-shaped lateral aspect of the foot indicates a (*pronated/supinated*) MTJ position.

supinated

18-61

Conversely, with MTJ pronation, the lateral aspect of the forefoot appears (*abducted/adducted*) on the lateral aspect of the rearfoot.

abducted

18-62

Sagittal plane subluxation during the propulsive period is indicative of abnormal STJ _____.

pronation

18-63

When the patient is walking toward the examiner, digital function during the propulsive period should be examined.

If the digits are pushing down against the floor, it is indicative of metatarsophalangeal joint (MPJ) stability and the gait is classified as propulsive. One way to judge digital pressure against the floor is to observe for momentary blanching of the toes during the propulsive period. If there is good momentary blanching of the digits, this is a good indication that the gait is propulsive.

18-64

If no blanching of the digits is observed and the digits cannot be seen pressing against the floor during the propulsive period, this would be classified as an _____ gait.

apropulsive

18-65

As is apparent, it takes much practice to perform the gait evaluation well. Like much of medicine, there is a big difference between reading about it and doing it.

Hopefully, this chapter will serve as a framework with which to begin.

This concludes the programmed portion of the book.

Questions

FRAME 18-2

1. Which of the following are measured in the patient's angle and base of gait?
   a. STJ neutral position
   b. RCSP
   c. tibial varum
   d. a and b
   e. b and c

FRAME 18-4

2. The normal angle of gait is between _____° and _____° abducted from the line of progression.
   a. 4, 7
   b. 7, 10
   c. 10, 13
   d. 13, 16
   e. 16, 19

FRAME 18-8

3. In order to perform the WB biomechanical measurements, the NWB calcaneal bisection may be used as long as the patient stands in the angle and base of gait.
   a. true
   b. false

FRAME 18-9

4. When the concavities above and below the lateral malleolus are equal, the:
   a. MTJ is maximally pronated
   b. MTJ is maximally supinated
   c. STJ is maximally pronated
   d. STJ is in its neutral position
   e. STJ is maximally supinated

FRAME 18-20

5. Tibial varum is measured with the patient in the:
   a. NCSP
   b. RCSP
   c. STJ neutral position
   d. natural rearfoot position
   e. orthopedic rearfoot position

FRAME 18-25

6. Before performing the gait evaluation, patients should have walked for a few minutes to slightly fatigue their muscles.
   a. true
   b. false

7. Sudden *internal* rotation of the knee just prior to heel contact may indicate:
   a. tight quadriceps
   b. tight medial hamstrings
   c. tight gastrocnemius
   d. tight soleus
   e. none of the above are correct

FRAME 18-30

8. When the knees are bowed in on a frontal plane and the legs are abducted relative to the thighs, it is called:
   a. external malleolar torsion
   b. internal malleolar torsion
   c. genu recurvatum
   d. genu varum
   e. genu valgum

FRAME 18-36

9. In *genu recurvatum,* the concavity faces anteriorly.
   a. true
   b. false

FRAME 18-39

10. Blanching of the digits during the propulsive period is indicative of a propulsive gait.
    a. true
    b. false

FRAME 18-63

Answers

1. e
2. b
3. b
4. d
5. a
6. a
7. b
8. e
9. a
10. a

APPENDIX 1

Signs and Symptoms Associated with Biomechanical Pathology in the Foot

---

Rearfoot Varus
1. Callus, plantar to the second metatarsal head
2. Callus, plantar to the fourth and fifth metatarsal heads
3. Tailor's bunion
4. Retrocalcaneal prominence (a.k.a. Haglund's deformity)
5. Ankle sprains of the inversion type
6. Adductovarus hammertoe deformities of the fourth and fifth digits
7. Mild hallux valgus deformity

Rearfoot Valgus
1. Callus, plantar to the second metatarsal head (note: not always present)
2. Fatigue of the muscles of the foot and leg
3. Pain at the plantar aspect of the medial longitudinal arch
4. Hallux valgus deformity

Forefoot Varus
1. Callus, plantar to the second, fourth, and/or fifth metatarsal heads
2. Fatigue in the muscles of the foot and leg
3. Tailor's bunion
4. Adductovarus hammertoe deformities of the fourth and fifth digits
5. Hallux valgus deformity

Forefoot Valgus/ Plantarflexed First Ray with Compensation by MTJ Longitudinal Axis Supination
1. Callus, plantar to the first and fifth metatarsal heads
2. Tibial sesamoiditis
3. Fatigue in the muscles of the foot and leg
4. Flexion contractures of the lesser digits
5. Lateral knee strain

Forefoot Valgus/ Plantarflexed First Ray with Compensation by Supination of the STJ and the MTJ Longitudinal and Oblique Axes
1. Callus, plantar to the first metatarsal head
2. Callus, plantar to the fourth and/or fifth metatarsal heads
3. Tibial sesamoiditis
4. Flexion contractures in the lesser digits
5. Lateral knee strain
6. Ankle sprains of the inversion type
7. Retrocalcaneal prominence (a.k.a. Haglund's deformity)
8. Pigeon-toed gait in children

Metatarsus Primus Elevatus	1. Callus, plantar to the second metatarsal head
2. Callus, plantar to the hallux proximal phalangeal head
3. Fatigue in the muscles of the foot and leg
4. Dorsal bunion at the first metatarsal head
5. Hallux limitus/rigidus deformity
Equinus Deformity in Children	1. Corn of the fifth toe
2. Adductovarus deformity of the fifth toe
3. Fatigue in the muscles of the foot and leg
4. "Growing pains" (cramps in the leg muscles)
5. Osteochondritis involving the navicular, cuneiform, or calcaneus
Equinus Deformity in Adults	1. Callus, plantar to the second metatarsal head
2. Adductovarus deformities of the fourth and fifth digits
3. Fatigue in the muscles of the foot and leg
4. Hallux valgus deformity

APPENDIX 2

Criteria for Normalcy in the Lower Extremity

Non-weightbearing

1. Malleolar torsion should be 13°–18° externally rotated.
2. Ankle joint dorsiflexion should be at least 10° with the knee extended.
3. Ankle joint plantarflexion should be at least 20°.
4. The total STJ ROM should be at least 8°–12°.
5. At the STJ neutral position, the calcaneal bisection should be parallel with the posterior distal one-third of the leg.
6. With regard to the MTJ, the plantar plane of the forefoot should be parallel with the plantar plane of the rearfoot when the foot is weightbearing and the MTJ is maximally pronated.
7. With regard to the first ray, there should be equal excursion in the dorsal and plantar directions (about 5 mm each way) from a level equal with the second metatarsal head when the STJ is in its neutral position and the MTJ is maximally pronated.
8. With regard to the fifth ray, there should be equal excursion in the dorsal and plantar directions from a level equal with the plane of the middle three metatarsals when the STJ is in its neutral position and the MTJ is maximally pronated.

Weightbearing

1. The distal one-third of the leg should be vertical.
2. The knee, ankle, and STJ should lie in transverse planes parallel to the supporting surfaces.
3. The STJ should rest in its neutral position.
4. A bisection of the posterior surface of the calcaneus should be vertical.
5. The MTJ should be locked in a maximally pronated position about both of its axes.
6. The plantar planes of the forefoot and the rearfoot should be parallel to each other and to the supporting surface.
7. The second, third, and fourth metatarsals should be completely dorsiflexed and the plantar surfaces of the metatarsal heads should describe a plane parallel to the supporting surface.
8. The first and fifth metatarsal heads should be in a position such that the plantar surfaces rest in a common transverse plane with the plantar surfaces of the middle three metatarsals.

APPENDIX 3

Effects in the Foot Secondary to Abnormal Propulsive STJ Pronation

1. Hallux abductovalgus, secondary to first ray and, therefore, first MPJ hypermobility
2. Medial bunion
3. Adductovarus contracture (hammertoe) of the lesser digits, especially the fourth and fifth digits
4. Reactive hyperkeratosis (corns) associated with adductovarus contracture
5. Hallux limits/Hallux rigidus, secondary to first ray and, therefore, first MPJ hypermobility
6. Tailor's bunion
7. Splayfoot
8. Fatigue of the muscles of the leg and foot
9. Weight overload of the lesser metatarsals
10. Hammertoe deformity

Glossary

Abducted	a position in which the foot or its distal part is rotated externally (parallel with a transverse plane) and in which the distal aspect of the foot or part faces away from the midline.
Abduction	movement on a transverse plane, away from the midline. Abduction of the foot occurs when the foot is rotated externally while remaining parallel to a transverse plane.
Abductory twist	a sudden abduction of the heel occurring just prior to toe off at the end of the propulsive period of gait.
Abductus	a fixed structural position in which the foot is held abducted.
Adducted	a position in which the foot or its distal part is rotated internally (parallel with a transverse plane) and in which the distal aspect of the foot or part faces toward the midline.
Adduction	movement on a transverse plane, toward the midline. Adduction of the foot occurs when the foot is rotated internally while remaining parallel to a transverse plane.
Adductovarus contracture	a contracture of the flexor tendons to the lesser digits which have not maintained a straight posterior vector relative to the toes. Instead, they have exerted a posterior-medial vector, thus causing the toes to be deformed and maintained in a plantarflexed and varus rotated position. This occurs secondary to abnormal propulsive STJ pronation and creates an adductovarus type of hammertoe.
Adductus	a fixed structural position in which the foot is held adducted.
Angle of gait	the angle which the feet assume relative to the body's line of progression during gait.
Ankle equinus	limitation of ankle joint dorsiflexion of less than 10° with the knee extended and flexed, due to a (usually) osseous blockage of dorsiflexion at the ankle joint. Usually, the Achilles tendon is not extremely tight at the end of the ankle dorsiflexory ROM.
Apropulsive gait	defined when there is no active propulsion by the digits during the propulsive period of gait.
Base of gait	the closest width between the malleoli during the midstance period of gait.
Bunion	a localized swelling at the first or fifth MPJ, caused by an inflammatory bursa or prominence or hyperostosis of the metatarsal head.
Closed Kinetic Chain (CKC)	the state of weightbearing; observed during the stance phase of the gait cycle.

Contact period	the first 30% of the stance phase of the gait cycle, lasting from heel strike of the same foot to toe off of the opposite foot. The contact period occurs after the swing phase and before the midstance period of the gait cycle.
Coronal plane	see Frontal plane.
Coxa	the hip or hip joint.
Coxa valga	a more vertical than normal orientation of the femoral head and neck.
Coxa vara	a more horizontal than normal orientation of the femoral head and neck.
Criteria for normalcy	biomechanical relationships which define the ideal biomechanical parameters in the foot and lower extremity.
Dorsiflexed	a position in which the foot is deviated in a sagittal body plane toward the tibia and above a transverse body plane passing through the heel of the foot. Alternately, a position in which a distal part of the foot is deviated in a sagittal plane above a transverse plane which runs through its proximal portion.
Dorsiflexion	movement of the foot toward the tibia in a sagittal plane.
Equinus	limitation of ankle joint dorsiflexion of less than 10° with the knee extended.
Eversion	motion of the foot—parallel to a frontal plane—that tilts the foot further away from the midline of the body.
Everted	a position of the foot in which it is tilted parallel with a frontal plane and in which the plantar surface faces away from the midline of the body and away from a transverse body plane.
First ray	the functional unit consisting of the first metatarsal and the first (medial) cuneiform.
Flexion contracture	a contracture of the flexor tendons to the lesser digits resulting in a toe which is maintained in a plantarflexed position at the PIPJ and DIPJ. The resulting deformity is a toe which is curled into a plantarflexed position—i.e., an exclusively sagittal plane deformity.
Forefoot adductus	a positional relationship between the metatarsus and the rearfoot in which the longitudinal axis of the metatarsus is adducted relative to the longitudinal axis of the rearfoot. This relationship changes based on the MTJ position.
Forefoot loading	that time beginning at the end of the contact period during which weight is transmitted into the forefoot, i.e., the forefoot becomes weight receptive.
Forefoot measuring device	an instrument used to measure the relationship of the plantar plane of the forefoot relative to the plantar plane of the rearfoot.
Forefoot rectus	a positional relationship between the metatarsus and the rearfoot in which the longitudinal axis of the metatarsus is parallel, or close to parallel, with the longitudinal axis of the rearfoot.
Forefoot supinatus	a relatively fixed, supinated position of the forefoot relative to the rearfoot with the STJ in its neutral position and the forefoot maximally pronated about both MTJ axes, caused by soft tissue adaptation. The MTJ ROM is typically decreased secondary to soft tissue contracture.

Forefoot valgus	a structural abnormality in which the plantar plane of the forefoot is everted relative to the plantar plane of the rearfoot when the STJ is in its neutral position and the forefoot is maximally pronated about both MTJ axes.
Forefoot varus	a structural abnormality in which the plantar plane of the forefoot is inverted relative to the plantar plane of the rearfoot when the STJ is in its neutral position and the forefoot is maximally pronated about both MTJ axes.
Frontal (coronal) plane	a vertical plane which is perpendicular to the sagittal plane and divides the body into front and back portions.
Gait cycle	that interval of time from heel strike of one foot to heel strike by the same foot at the next step.
Gastocnemius equinus	a limitation of ankle joint dorsiflexion of less than 10° which is only observed with the knee extended. The Achilles tendon becomes tight at the end of the ankle dorsiflexory ROM with the knee extended. A normal amount of ankle dorsiflexion is observed with the knee flexed.
Genu	the knee.
Genu recurvatum	hyperextension of the knee with the concavity facing anteriorly.
Genu valgum	"knock-knees"; a deformity in which the legs are abducted relative to the thighs. The knees are bowed in toward each other on a frontal plane.
Genu varum	"bow-legs"; a deformity in which the knees are bowed out away from each other on a frontal plane.
Goniometer	an instrument used for measuring angles (a.k.a. tractograph).
Gravity goniometer	a calipered instrument with a weighted, freely swinging needle mounted on a 360° scale used to measure angles.
Hallux abductovalgus (HAV)	a relatively fixed abnormality in which the hallux is maintained in a state of valgus rotation and is abducted from the midline of the body at the first MPJ. (Sometimes, an abnormal abducted position may also exist at the hallux IPJ.)
Hallux limitus or hallux rigidus	frequently used interchangeably, these terms refer to a painful limitation of dorsiflexion at the first MPJ. A limitation in plantarflexion may exist concomitantly.
Hallux valgus	see Hallux abductovalgus.
Head tilt	angular deviation of the head from a midsagittal plane.
Horizontal plane	see Transverse plane.
Hypermobility	movement in a segment or part which should be stable or fixed when stress is applied.
Inversion	motion of the foot parallel with a frontal plane that tilts the foot more toward the midline of the body.
Inverted	a position of the foot in which it is tilted parallel with a frontal plane and in which the plantar surface of the foot faces toward the midline of the body and away from a transverse body plane.
Malleolar torsion	the amount of rotation from the frontal plane of a line connecting the medial and lateral malleoli. This is an index of tibial torsion—i.e., growth in the transverse plane.

Metatarsus adductus	the fixed structural angular relationship between the metatarsus and the lesser tarsus.
Metatarsus primus elevatus	a structural abnormality in which the first ray has more dorsiflexion than plantarflexion. This is observed as the ROM of the first metatarsal head —relative to the plane of the second through fifth metatarsal heads— with the STJ in its neutral position and the forefoot maximally pronated about both MTJ axes.
Midstance period	the part of the stance phase which occurs between toe off of the opposite foot and heel lift of the same foot. The midstance period occurs between the contact and propulsive periods of the stance phase of the gait cycle and represents about 40% of the stance phase.
Neutral Calcaneal Stance Position (NCSP)	the angular relationship of the calcaneus relative to the ground with the STJ in its neutral position and the patient standing in the angle and base of gait.
Neutral Position (NP)	with regard to the STJ, that position in an ideal foot which separates a pronated position from a supinated position. When the STJ is in its neutral position, the foot is not in a supinated or pronated position. Additionally, in the normal foot, there is twice as much supinatory motion as there is pronatory motion from the STJ neutral position.
Open Kinetic Chain (OKC)	the state of non-weightbearing; observed during the swing phase of the gait cycle.
Paresis	partial or incomplete paralysis.
Paretic	relating to or suffering from paresis.
Plantarflexed	a position in which the foot is deviated in a sagittal body plane away from the tibia and below a transverse plane passing through the heel of the foot. Alternately, a position in which a distal part of the foot is deviated in a sagittal plane below a transverse plane which runs through its proximal portion.
Plantarflexed first ray	a structural abnormality in which the first ray has more plantarflexion than dorsiflexion. This is observed as the ROM of the first metatarsal head relative to the plane of the second through fifth metatarsal heads; the STJ is in its neutral position, and the forefoot is maximally pronated about both MTJ axes.
Plantarflexion	movement of the foot away from the tibia in a sagittal plane.
Pronated	a position of the foot in which it is simultaneously abducted, dorsiflexed, and everted.
Pronation	a triplane motion of the foot composed of abduction, dorsiflexion, and eversion.
Propulsive gait	defined when there is active digital propulsion during the propulsive period of gait.
Propulsive period	that part of the stance phase of the gait cycle which occurs between heel lift and toe off of the same foot. The propulsive period occurs after the midstance period and before the beginning of the swing phase of the gait cycle. The propulsive period represents about 30% of the stance phase of the gait cycle.
Ray	a functional metatarsal unit. For the medial three rays, this consists of the metatarsal and its respective cuneiform. For the fourth and fifth rays, this consists of the metatarsal only.

Rearfoot valgus	a condition in which the calcaneus is everted relative to the ground with the STJ in its neutral position.
Rearfoot varus	a condition in which the calcaneus is inverted relative to the ground with the STJ in its neutral position.
Relaxed Calcaneal Stance Position (RCSP)	the angular relationship of the calcaneus relative to the ground with the patient standing relaxed in the angle and base of gait.
Sagittal plane	an anterior-posterior plane which divides the body into right and left portions.
Scoliosis	abnormal frontal plane curvature of the spine.
Soleus equinus	a limitation of ankle joint dorsiflexion of less than 10° with the knee extended and flexed which is caused by a short soleus muscle or tendon. The Achilles tendon becomes extremely tight at the end of the ankle dorsiflexory ROM.
Spasm	an involuntary muscle contraction or increased muscular tension and shortness which cannot be released voluntarily and which prevents lengthening of the muscles involved.
Stance phase	the weightbearing portion of the gait cycle which occurs between heel strike and toe off of the same foot. The stance phase comprises about 60% of the total gait cycle. The three subdivisions of the stance phase are the contact, midstance, and propulsive periods.
Subluxation	a state of partial or incomplete dislocation.
Subtalar valgus	a STJ neutral position in which the calcaneal bisection is everted relative to the longitudinal bisection of the distal one-third of the leg.
Subtalar varus	a STJ neutral position in which the calcaneal bisection is inverted relative to the longitudinal bisection of the distal one-third of the leg.
Supinated	a position of the foot in which it is simultaneously adducted, plantarflexed, and inverted.
Supination	a triplane motion of the foot which is composed of adduction, plantarflexion, and inversion.
Swing phase	the non-weight-bearing portion of the gait cycle which occurs between toe off and heel strike of the same foot. The swing phase comprises about 40% of the total gait cycle.
Tailor's bunion	a localized swelling at the fifth MPJ caused by an inflammatory bursa or prominence or hyperostosis of the fifth metatarsal head.
Talipes calcaneus	a fixed structural position in which the foot is maintained in a plantarflexed position.
Talipes equinus	a fixed structural position in which the foot is maintained in a dorsiflexed position.
Tarsal coalition	the abnormal union (osseous, cartilagenous, or fibrous) of two or more tarsal bones.
Tibial valgum	an abnormal frontal plane orientation of the tibia in which the distal aspect of the tibia is everted relative to the proximal aspect of the tibia with the patient standing in the angle and base of gait with the foot maintained in the NCSP.
Tibial varum	an abnormal frontal plane orientation of the tibia in which the distal aspect of the tibia is inverted relative to the proximal aspect of the tibia

	with the patient standing in the angle and base of gait with the foot maintained in the NCSP.
Tonic spasm	a continuous involuntary muscle contraction.
Tractograph	an instrument used for measuring angles (a.k.a. goniometer).
Transverse (horizontal) plane	a plane which is perpendicular to the frontal and sagittal planes and which divides the body into upper and lower portions.
Triplane motion	motion which occurs about a triplane axis and which is not parallel to any of the body planes.
Valgus	a fixed structural position in which the foot is maintained in an everted position.
Varus	a fixed structural position in which the foot is maintained in an inverted position.

Index

Abducted, 8, 11
Abduction, 3, 6, 8, 17, 137
Abnormal shearing forces, 48
Achilles tendon, 216
Adducted, 9–11
Adduction, 4, 6, 8, 10, 17, 137
Adductovarus
   contracture, 183
   hammertoe, 179
Angle of gait, 100–101, 238
Ankle
   dorsiflexion, 214–216
   equinus, 215–216
Anterior tibial, 82, 98, 154
Apropulsive, 198, 209, 249
Axis, 15–18

Base of gait, 100–101, 238
Biomechanical examination, 213–234
Bisection
   calcaneal, 144, 220
   leg, 74

Calcaneus, 52–54, 62–63, 66, 220, 222
   eversion, 74
   forefoot varus, 171
   index of subtalar joint motion, 69
   inversion, 74, 248
   parallel, 99
   relaxed calcaneal stance position, 105
   weightbearing measurements, 239
Calluses, 48
Central three rays, 32–34
Charcot-Marie-Tooth disease, 83
CKC (*see* Closed kinetic chain)
Closed kinetic chain, 52–55
Contact period
   calcaneus, 247
   definition, 44–46, 124
   forefoot, 163
   midtarsal joint, 152, 158
   rearfoot, 156
   subtalar joint, 62, 126, 247
Coxa valga, 246
Coxa vara, 245

Degenerative joint disease, 244
Dorsiflexed, 5, 8, 11
Dorsiflexion, 4–6, 8, 16–17, 137, 194, 197
   restriction, 216

Equinus state, 215
Equinus-type foot, 129–131

Eversion, 6–8, 16–17, 70, 138, 194
Everted, 8–9
Extensor digitorum longus, 83, 98, 154

Fifth ray axis, 31, 196
First ray axis, 21–23, 25, 29, 31, 137
   hypermobility, 190
   motion, 188, 195
   range of motion, 189, 228, 230–231
Flexor digitorum longus
   muscle, 197–198
   tendons, 183
Forefoot, 155, 158, 161–163
   adductus, 193, 195
   loading, 42, 155–157
   measuring device, 145, 227
   rectus, 193, 210
   supinatus, 169–170, 173, 178–179
   to rearfoot relationship, 226–227, 231
   valgus, 166–167, 179–182, 202–205, 207, 228
   varus, 166–179, 227
      hyperkeratotic accumulations, 177–178
Frontal plane, 1–2, 6–8, 70, 218, 242
   motion, 136, 138–139, 248

Gait cycle, 41–48, 59, 123–131, 237
   evaluation, 244
Gastrocnemius, 82–84, 98, 215–216
   equinus, 216–217
Gastrocsoleus, 98
Genu valgum configuration, 176, 245–246
Genu varum, 246
Genu recurvatum, 246
Goniometer, 144–145, 224, 227, 232, 241, 243
   (*see also* Tractograph)

Hallux
   abductovalgus, 191–193, 195
   limitus, 191–193, 195, 209–210
   rigidus, 191–193, 209–210
   valgus, 179
Head tilt, 244
Heel
   lift, 42, 46, 63, 158
   strike, 42, 60, 63, 65, 123, 126, 156
Hyperkeratosis
   forefoot valgus, 183
   metatarsus primus elevatus, 208
Hypermobility, 48, 127, 191, 210

Iliac crest height, 245
Interphalangeal joint axis, 31–32, 34
Inversion, 6–8, 16–17, 138, 194
Inverted, 7–8
IPJ (*see* Interphalangeal joint)

Kinetic chain, 51
Knee strain, 178, 183

Lateral malleolus, 219
Lateral malleoli, 232
Limb length discrepancy, 244
Long digital flexors, 82, 84, 98

Malleolar torsion, 231–232, 234
Medial hamstrings, 245
Medial malleoli, 232
Metatarsal heads, 127
Metatarsophalangeal joint, 191
   axis, 31–34
Metatarsus primus elevatus, 206–210, 230
Midstance period
   calcaneus, 54
   definition, 44–46, 124
   first ray, 194, 207
   midtarsal joint, 158
   subtalar joint, 65, 126, 152, 160–161, 248–249
Midtarsal joint
   dorsiflexion, 160
   forefoot valgus, 180
   forefoot varus, 174, 176
   plantarflexion, 160
   position, 145, 165, 225
   pronation, 141, 153–154, 171, 179, 249
   range of motion, 141–143, 145, 149–152, 157, 169–170
   subluxation, 192
   supination, 153–154
Midtarsal joint axis
   longitudinal, 34–35, 37, 135–139, 154–163, 180–182, 205, 225
   oblique, 34–37, 135, 137–139, 145, 154–156, 158–161, 163, 180
Midtarsal joint deformities (*see* Forefoot valgus, forefoot varus)
Midtarsal joints
   calcaneocuboid, 139
   talonavicular, 139
Mobile adaptor, 61
MPJ (*see* Metatarsophalangeal joint)
MTJ (*see* Midtarsal joint)

NCSP (*see* Neutral calcaneal stance position)
Neuromuscular disease, 244
Neutral calcaneal stance position, 101–103, 106, 237, 239–243
Neurologic deficit, 244
Neutral position
  subtalar joint, 60, 70–71
Non-weightbearing
  exam, 241
NWB (*see* Non-weightbearing)

OKC (*see* Open kinetic chain)
Open kinetic chain, 52, 54, 59, 65

Peroneal muscles, 159, 162
Peroneus
  brevis, 83–84, 98
  longus, 23, 83, 98, 205
  tertius, 83, 98, 154
Plane motion, 2–12 (*see also* Abduction, Adduction, Dorsiflexion, Eversion, Inversion, Plantarflexion, Pronation, Supination, Talipes calcaneus, Talipes equinus)
Plane positions, 5–7, 9–12 (*see also* Abducted, Adducted, Dorsiflexed, Everted, Inverted, Plantarflexed, Valgus, Varus)
Planes, 1–8 (*see also* Frontal, Plantar, Sagittal, Transverse)
Plantarflexed, 5, 8–9, 11–12
  cuboid (*see* Forefoot varus)
  fifth metatarsal (*see* Forefoot varus)
  first ray, 202–206, 208–209
Plantarflexion, 4–5, 16–17, 137, 194, 197
Plantar plane
  forefoot, 140, 142–144, 226
  rearfoot, 140, 142–144, 226
Posterior tibial, 82, 84, 98
Pronation, 8–10, 12, 18, 26–28, 43
  adduction of the talus, 64
  chronic, 182
  rearfoot, 155
  subtalar joint, 60, 65
Propulsive period
  definition, 44–46, 124, 160
  first ray, 190, 193–195, 207
  forefoot, 162, 175
  hypermobility, 210
  midtarsal joint, 152
  peroneal muscles, 159
  subtalar joint, 63, 66, 126, 158–160, 214, 217, 248–249

tibia, 66
toes, 197–198

RCSP (*see* Relaxed calcaneal stance position)
Rearfoot, 158, 161
  eversion, 157
  pronation, 155–156
  valgus, 90, 93–94, 102, 106, 130–131
    tibial varum, 105
    case history, 119, 121
  varus, 90–91, 93–94, 99–100, 102–103, 106, 128–129, 181
    case history, 116–118, 122
    compensated, 105
    propulsive period, 130–131
    relaxed calcaneal stance position, 104
    subtalar joint, 143
Relaxed calcaneal stance position, 103–104, 106, 237, 241–242
Retrocalcaneal prominence, 122
ROM (*see* Range of motion)

Sagittal plane
  definition, 1–4
  hallux limitus, 193
  midtarsal joint, 138–139
  subluxation, 249
  subtalar joint, 81, 98
  talipes equinus, 12
Scoliosis, 244
Soleus, 82
Soleus equinus, 215–216
Stance phase
  calcaneus, 54
  definition, 124
  forefoot varus, 174
  gait cycle, 41, 43–46
  midtarsal joint, 155
  midtarsal joint oblique axis, 158
  subtalar joint, 176
STJ (*see* Subtalar joint)
Subluxations, 48, 127, 249
Subtalar joint, 24–26, 47–48, 51, 161
  axis, 26–31, 63, 81–82, 97
  forefoot valgus, 180
  forefoot varus, 175
  function, 246
  gait cycle, 59–66, 157
  motion, 69–77, 125
  neutral position, 85–87, 99, 103, 144, 172, 179, 219, 224, 229–230, 240
  pronation, 106, 118–119, 122, 126, 129, 131, 139, 150–151, 153, 158, 171, 173–174, 178–179,

181, 183, 190–191, 194, 210, 214, 217, 232, 248
  range of motion, 172–173, 218, 221, 224–225
  rearfoot valgus, 105
  supination, 98, 126, 128–129, 131, 142, 144, 150, 152–153, 158, 160–162, 180–181, 206, 222, 248
Subtalar valgus, 87, 89–90, 93–94
Subtalar varus, 87–89, 93–94, 99
  varus torsion, 89
Supination, 8–10, 12, 18, 26–28, 43, 53–54, 225
  Open kinetic chain, 60, 65
Swing phase, 41–43, 46, 54, 59–60, 62, 125, 153
  first ray, 194–195
  forefoot, 162
  pronation, 126
  supination, 126
Symmetrical rotation, 244
Synchondrosis, 94
Syndesmosis, 94
Synostosis, 94

Tailor's bunion, 179
Talipes calcaneus, 11–12
Talipes equinus, 12
Talonavicular joint, 219
Talus, 53, 61–63, 66, 232
Tarsal coalition, 92–94, 130–131
Tibia, 232, 242
Tibial rotations, 55, 66
  position, 246
  torsion, 231
  valgum, 100–101, 121, 237
  varum, 91, 93, 100–101, 103, 106, 237, 242–243
TNJ (*see* Talonavicular joint)
Toe off, 42, 248
Tractograph, 144–145 (*see also* Goniometer)
Transverse plane
  closed kinetic chain, 66
  definition, 1–5
  eversion, 7
  first ray axis, 21
  hallux abductovalgus, 193
  inversion, 8
  malleolar torsion, 231
  midtarsal joint oblique axis, 138–139
  subtalar joint, 98
  subtalar joint axis, 81
  talipes equinus, 11–12
Triplane motion, 136

Valgus, 11–12
Varus, 11–12